Precursors of
Gastric Cancer

Precursors of Gastric Cancer

Edited by
Si-Chun Ming, M.D.

Professor, Department of Pathology,
Temple University School of Medicine

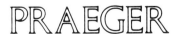

PRAEGER SPECIAL STUDIES • PRAEGER SCIENTIFIC

New York • Philadelphia • Eastbourne, UK
Toronto • Hong Kong • Tokyo • Sydney

Library of Congress Cataloging in Publication Data

Main entry under title:

Precursors of gastric cancer.

  Bibliography: p.
  Includes index.
    1. Stomach—Cancer—Etiology—Congresses. 2. Stomach—
Diseases—Complications and sequelae—Congresses.
I. Ming, Si-Chun. [DNLM: 1. Precancerous conditions—
Congresses. 2. Stomach neoplasms—Congresses. WI 320
P923 1982]
RC280.S8P74   1984   616.99'43307   83-27025
ISBN 0-03-063969-7 (alk. paper)

Published in 1984 by Praeger Publishers
CBS Educational and Professional Publishing,
a Division of CBS Inc.
521 Fifth Avenue, New York, NY 10175 USA

© 1984 by Praeger Publishers

456789 052 9876545321

Printed in the United States of America
on acid-free paper

PREFACE

In view of the worldwide prevalence of gastric cancer and its grave morbidity and mortality, there have been increasing efforts in recent years to identify precancerous lesions of the stomach in order to detect gastric cancer at the initial stage by follow-up studies or even possibly to prevent cancer development by proper management of these lesions. These efforts are facilitated by the use of endoscopic biopsy and subsequent pathological evaluation. Emphasis on this aspect of the study of gastric cancer has resulted in the publication of several classification systems for gastric dysplasia, which is considered to be the essential feature of premalignant changes. In order to reach a unified concept and to establish the criteria for the pathological diagnosis of gastric dysplasia, a three-day Workshop on Gastric Dysplasia and Related Lesions was held in June 1982 at S. Miniato near Florence, Italy, under the joint sponsorship of the International Study Group on Gastric Cancer (Executive Officer, Prof. Massimo Crespi) and the Institute of Anatomy and Histologic Pathology of the University of Florence (Director, Prof. Giancarlo Zampi).

At the workshop representative as well as controversial microscopic slides of various gastric lesions were reviewed and discussed in order to identify criteria and to evaluate the significance of various grades of abnormality. In addition, research data were presented relating dysplasia to various precancerous clinical and pathological conditions and, in turn, the latter to gastric cancer. This volume is composed of expanded and updated versions of the topics discussed at the workshop as well as other related topics not formally presented. Therefore, it contains the current opinions on the precursors of gastric cancer. The expressed views are those of the individual investigators, however, and not the group as a whole. They should be valuable to both pathologists and clinicians in their evaluation of patients who may potentially develop a gastric cancer.

Sincere gratitude is hereby expressed toward all the authors who actively participated in the workshop and enthusiastically contributed their expertise and knowledge to this volume. Special thanks are due to Prof. Zampi for his sponsorship of the workshop, which was held in a magnificent setting provided by the University of Florence.

Si-Chun Ming, M.D.

LIST OF CONTRIBUTORS

Christine Amat, M.D. Service d'Anatomie et de Cytologie Pathologiques, Hopital Broussais, 75674 Paris Cedex 14, France.

Attila Bajtai, M.D. Department of Pathological Anatomy, Postgraduate Medical School, Budapest XIII, Szabolc u. 35, Hungary.

Jean Pierre Camilleri, M.D. Service d'Anatomie et de Cytologie Pathologiques, Hopital Broussais, 75674 Paris Cedex 14, France.

M. L. Carcangiu, M.D. Istituto di Anatomia e Istologia Patologica, Universita di Firenze, 50134 Firenze, Italy.

Walter Carson, M.D. Department of Pathology, Municipal Hospital, Kulmbacher Str. 23, D-8580, Bayreuth, F.R.G.

Rodolfo Cheli, M.D. Chief, Divisione di Gastroenterologia, Ospedale S. Martino, 16132 Genova, Italy.

Pelayo Correa, M.D. Professor, Department of Pathology, Louisiana State University Medical Center, 1901 Perdido Street, New Orleans, Louisiana 70112, U.S.A.

Masashi Daibo, M.D. First Histopathology Section, Pathology Division, National Cancer Center Research Institute, Tsukiji 5-Chome, Chuo-ku, Tokyo, Japan.

Harro Eidt, M.D. Department of Pathology, Municipal Hospital, Kulmbacher Str. 23, D-8580 Bayreuth, F.R.G.

Kurt Elster, M.D. Professor, Department of Pathology, Municipal Hospital, Kulmbacher Str. 23, D-8580 Bayreuth, F.R.G.

Adel Gad, M.D., Ph.D. Department of Clinical Pathology and Cytology, Falun Hospital, S-791 82 Falun, Sweden.

Attilio Giacosa, M.D. Assistant, Divisione di Gastroenterologia, Ospedale S. Martino, 16132 Genova, Italy.

Ilkka P. T. Häkkinen, M.D. Department of Pathology, University of Turku, SF-20520, Turku 52, Finland.

Takuji Hayashi, M.D. Department of Pathology, Kuakini Medical Center, 347 North Kuakini Street, Honolulu, Hawaii 96817, U.S.A.

Takeshi Hirayama, M.D. Chief, Epidemiology Division, National Cancer Center Research Institute, Tsukiji 5-Chome, Chuo-ku, Tokyo, Japan.

Teruyuki Hirota, M.D. Head, First Histopathology Section, Pathology Division, National Cancer Center Research Institute, Tsukiji 5-Chome, Chuo-ku, Tokyo, Japan.

Masayuki Itabashi, M.D. Chief Researcher, First Histopathology Section, Pathology Division, National Cancer Center Research Institute, Tsukiji 5-Chome, Chuo-ku, Tokyo, Japan.

J. Juhász, M.D. Professor and Head, Department of Pathological Anatomy, Postgraduate Medical School, Budapest XIII, Szabolc u. 35, Hungary.

Osmo H. Järvi, M.D. Professor, Department of Pathology, University of Turku, SF-20520 Turku 52, Finland.

Jeremy R. Jass, B.Sc., M.B., B.S. Senior Lecturer and Honorary Consultant, Department of Histopathology, Westminster Medical School, 17 Horseferry Road, London SW1p 2AR, U.K.

Hisazo Kitaoka, M.D. Chief, Surgery Division, National Cancer Center Hospital, Tsukiji 5-Chome, Chuo-ku, Tokyo, Japan.

Norio Matsukura, M.D. Biochemistry Division, National Cancer Center Research Institute, Tsukiji 5-Chome, Chuo-ku, Tokyo, Japan.

Si-Chun Ming, M.D. Professor, Department of Pathology, Temple University School of Medicine, 3400 North Broad Street, Philadelphia, Pennsylvania 19140, U.S.A.

Georges Molas, M.D. Service d'Anatomie et de Cytologie Pathologiques, Hopital Beaujon, 92118 Clichy Cedex, France.

Johannes Myren, M.D. Department of Internal Medicine 9, Ulleval University Hospital, Oslo 1, Norway.

Takeo Nagayo, M.D. Director, Aichi Cancer Center Research Institute, Chikusa-ku, Nagoya, Japan.

Wolfgang Oehlert, M.D. Professor and Director, Hepato-Gastro-Enterologie, Pathologisches Institut, Klinikum der Albert-Ludwigs-Universitat, Albertstr. 19, 78 Freiburg, F.R.G.

Toshio Okada, M.D. Researcher, First Histopathology Section, Pathology Division, National Cancer Center Research Institute, Tsukiji 5-Chome, Chuo-ku, Tokyo, Japan.

Magne Osnes, M.D. Gastroenterological Section, Department of Internal Medicine 9, Ulleval University Hospital, Oslo 1, Norway.

Alessandro Perasso, M.D. Assistant, Divisione di Gastroenterologia, Ospedale S. Martino, 16132 Genova, Italy.

Francois Potet, M.D. Service d'Anatomie et de Cytologie Pathologiques, Hospital Beaujon, 92118 Clichy Cedex, France.

Ryozo Sano, M.D.* First Histopathology Section, Pathology Division, National Cancer Center Research Institute, Tsukiji 5-Chome, Chuo-ku, Tokyo, Japan.

Arne Serck-Hanssen, M.D. Department of Pathology, Ulleval University Hospital, Oslo 1, Norway.

Grant N. Stemmermann, M.D. Director, Department of Pathology, Kuakini Medical Center, 347 North Kuakini Street, Honolulu, Hawaii 96817, U.S.A.

Manfred Stolte, M.D. Professor, Department of Pathology, Municipal Hospital, Kulmbacher Str. 23, D-8580 Bayreuth, F.R.G.

Stephanie Teruya, B.Sc. Department of Pathology, Kuakini Medical Center, 347 North Kuakini Street, Honolulu, Hawaii 96817, U.S.A.

Hitoshi Yoshida, M.D. First Histopathology Section, Pathology Division, National Cancer Center Research Institute, Tsukiji 5-Chome, Chuo-ku, Tokyo, Japan.

Giancarlo Zampi, M.D. Istituto di Anatomia e Istologia Pathologica, Universita di Firenze, Firenze, Italy.

Yinchang Zhang, M.D. Chief, Department of Cancer Research, China Medical College, Shenyang, People's Republic of China.

*Deceased.

CONTENTS

INTRODUCTION

1 INTRODUCTION

S.-C. Ming

Gastric cancer is a deadly disease and carries with it a very high mortality rate. The main reason appears to be late diagnosis. For instance, among 1,134 patients staged by Kennedy (1), only 32 were in the T_1 stage (carcinoma limited to the gastric mucosa). A major effort was undertaken for the early diagnosis of gastric carcinoma. It met with notable success in high-risk countries such as Japan, where a mass survey detected a high percentage of patients with early gastric carcinoma, with a corresponding improvement in the survival rate (2). In other countries, such as the United States, early diagnosis of gastric cancer among hospital patients has not increased dramatically in spite of common usage of gastroscopy as a routine diagnostic tool; the overall survival rate for gastric cancer remains as low as before (3, 4). Thus, the contribution from early diagnosis in the management of gastric cancer appears to have reached a plateau.

It has long been recognized that gastric cancer occurs more frequently in certain conditions. As long ago as 1929, Hurst (5) recognized chronic atrophic gastritis, chronic ulcer, adenoma, and polyp as precursors of gastric carcinoma. Progress has been made continuously in relating these conditions to the development of gastric carcinoma. In addition to the conditions mentioned above, pernicious anemia is a long-recognized precancerous condition, because of severe chronic atrophic gastritis. Intestinal metaplasia is another precancerous condition that has received particular attention in recent years

Table 1-1. Precursors of Gastric Cancer

Chronic atrophic gastritis
Intestinal metaplasia
Chronic gastric ulcer
Epithelial polyps of stomach
Adenoma
Hyperplastic polyp
Generalized polyposis
Postresection gastric stump
Mucosal hyperplasia
Menetrier's disease

because of the recognition of the complexity of the metaplastic epithelium. Increased incidence of gastric cancer has also been reported in other conditions. (Table 1-1).

It has been suggested that precursors of gastric cancer can be divided into two categories: precancerous conditions and precancerous lesions (6). Precancerous conditions are clinical entities in which there is increased incidence of gastric cancer development, whereas precancerous lesions are pathological lesions from which gastric carcinoma develops. In many precancerous conditions, the actual precancerous lesion is dysplasia of the epithelium that may be metaplastic or nonmetaplastic. Thus, chronic atrophic gastritis is a precancerous condition, and the dysplastic epithelium in the atrophic mucosa is a precancerous lesion. In adenoma, the cells are already dysplastic; therefore, adenoma itself is a precancerous lesion.

Only recently, dysplasia of the gastric epithelium has become a subject of systematic investigation. Since dysplasia is a tissue-specific alteration, pathologists are responsible for defining it in pathological terms. On the other hand, the significance of dysplasia lies in its clinical implication. There must be, therefore, close clinicopathological correlative studies.

In this volume the current views on various precursors of gastric cancer are presented. These views of individual authors are based on their own experience, and not the collective views of the group. The chapters are grouped into major categories. It is evident, however, that there are unavoidable overlaps, as the same tissue change may occur in several conditions.

REFERENCES

1. Kennedy, B. J. TNM classification for stomach cancer. *Cancer* 26 (1970):971–983.
2. Ariga, K., and Takahashi, K. Gastric mass survey. *Gann Monogr. Cancer Res.* 18 (1976):99–103.

3. Dupont, B. J., Jr., and Cohn, I., Jr. Gastric carcinoma. *Curr. Prob. Cancer* 4 (1980):1–46.
4. Bizer, L. S. Adenocarcinoma of the stomach—Current results of treatment. *Cancer* 51 (1983):743–745.
5. Hurst, A. F. Precursors of carcinoma of the stomach. *Lancet* 2 (1929):1023.
6. Morson, B. C., Sobin, L. H., Grundmann, E., Johansen, A., Nagayo, T., and Serck-Hanssen, A. Precancerous conditions and epithelial dysplasia in the stomach. *J. Clin. Pathol.* 33 (1980):711–721.

II DYSPLASIA OF GASTRIC EPITHELIUM

2 PATHOLOGICAL FEATURES AND SIGNIFICANCE OF GASTRIC DYSPLASIA

S.-C. Ming

The low survival rate of gastric carcinoma has been offset by the diagnosis of early gastric cancer in increasing numbers of patients as the acuity of endoscopic diagnosis advances. Gastroscopy is now a commonly practiced procedure, and gastroscopic biopsies are common pathological specimens. Consequently, gastric dysplasia is now often encountered and has become a major concern for pathologists as well as clinicians. It implies possible, even imminent, malignant change, sometimes without a sound basis, and poses a difficult therapeutic problem. It is therefore of practical importance to clarify the meaning and significance of gastric dysplasia and to define clearly its pathological criteria, so that proper management and follow-up studies may be instituted.

Dysplasia means abnormality of development. In pathology this term is applied to cellular abnormalities, such as abnormal cytological features and organizational derangements. When used in the context of carcinogenesis, dysplasia denotes serious cellular changes that, in time, lead to the development of cancer. It can occur in several precancerous conditions. In the case of the stomach, several precancerous conditions have long been recognized (see Table 1-1). Although gastric dysplasia has also been recognized for some time, systematic study of this lesion is a rather recent undertaking, that is, since 1979 (1–9).

Dysplasia as a precancerous lesion has been applied to several organs, notably the uterine cervix. The status of understanding with regard to gastric dysplasia corresponds to that of cervical dysplasia in the early period of investigation, when the diagnostic criteria and the relationship to cancer were still unsettled. Thus, the reports on gastric dysplasia have dwelt largely on classification methods and have introduced a number of terms to describe different types and gradations of pathological alterations. However, there have been very few reports dealing with the development of cancer in the dysplastic epithelium.

If one considers all forms of mucosal abnormality of the stomach as dysplastic, four gradations of dysplasia, grades 1 to 4 in order of increasing degree of abnormality, can be recognized (6). In terms of their potential for malignant transformation, it has been assumed that the greater the abnormality, the likelier is the possibility of malignant change. In other words, only the high grades of dysplasia may be closely related to cancer. This seems indeed the case when comparing the incidence of dysplasia in stomachs with carcinoma with that in stomachs with benign diseases (6). On the other hand, follow-up studies carried out by Oehlert (4) demonstrated a high regression rate even for high-grade dysplasia. He did find, however, malignant change in 8.7 percent of cases with persistent high-grade dysplasia for more than 3 years.

In order to unify the concept of gastric dysplasia and agree on the criteria for its pathological diagnosis, the Pathology Panel of the International Study Group on Gastric Cancer (ISGGC; members are A. Bajtai, P. Correa, K. Elster, O. Järvi, S. Ming (Chairman), N. Munoz, T. Nagayo, and G. Stemmermann) reviewed 93 microslides representative of varying degrees of gastric abnormalities. The members' views were then discussed at a workshop, under the auspices of the Department of Histopathology of the University of Florence (Director, Prof. G. Zampi), held at San Miniato, Italy, during June 1982. Most contributors to this volume also participated in the discussion and offered many valuable views. Some opinions of the panel members are included, and the pathological features of various types of epithelial changes are presented in this chapter.

SIGNIFICANCE OF GASTRIC DYSPLASIA

The significance of gastric dysplasia lies in its precancerous nature, which is indicated by its frequent association with cancer and the subsequent development of cancer in the same general region of the stomach.

Severe dysplasia has been found in a much higher percentage of cancerous stomachs than of benign stomachs (6, 10), with about equal involvement of metaplastic and nonmetaplastic glands (11). Furthermore, high grades of dysplasia were found more frequently in association with the expanding type of gastric cancer than with the infiltrative type (6). Close association has also been noted between dysplasia and the intestinal type of carcinoma but not between dysplasia and the diffuse type of carcinoma (12, 13). It must be recognized, however, that the exact relationship between gastric dysplasia and cancer is difficult to evaluate from these observations. Although it is possible that dysplasia preceded the cancer, it is also possible that they merely coexisted, either independently or under the same etiologic influence. Only the development of cancer in the dysplastic epithelium gives affirmative indication of the precancerous nature of gastric dysplasia. Such evidence has been found in adenomas of the stomach, which are composed of dysplastic cells and have a high incidence of malignant change (see Chapter 18). Under other circumstances, such as chronic atrophic gastritis, the degree of dysplasia varies greatly, and there are very few follow-up studies detailing the incidence of cancer development.

Siurala (14) followed patients with chronic atrophic gastritis for about 20 years. Ten percent developed carcinoma and 37 percent dysplasia, while these figures were 0.6 and 6 percent, respectively, in the control cases. Similar observations were made for stomach stumps after partial gastrectomy (15). These studies again suggest but do not establish the causal relationship between dysplasia and cancer. Oehlert et al. (5) actually followed the evolution of dysplastic epithelium by periodic biopsies. Although there is the obvious difficulty of ensuring that the biopsies came from the same focus, the results are revealing: Carcinoma developed in 8.7 percent of cases whose dysplasia had persisted for more than 3 years. At the same time, it was discovered that dysplasia often regresses, but the rate of regression diminishes as the duration of the dysplasia increases.

These studies support the long-held view that dysplasia is a precancerous lesion and that carcinoma will develop in the dysplastic epithelium if the dysplastic changes persist for a long time. It is clear, however, that definitive data are lacking, and there is a need for more prospective studies.

CLASSIFICATION OF ABNORMAL GASTRIC EPITHELIUM

Dysplasia has been graded according to the degree of abnormalities. The normal gastric epithelium is a rather quiescent organ. It is composed of mature, well-differentiated cells, with a proliferating zone normally residing at the neck region of the glands (16) where occasional mitosis may be seen.

If one takes the broad view that any deviation of the gastric epithelium from normal is dysplastic, then dysplasia would include regenerative changes at the edge of a healing ulcer, the mature but irregularly dilated foveolae in a hyperplastic polyp, and other proliferative cells of any benign lesion. In most systems regenerative or inflammatory changes are excluded, and dysplasia is divided usually into three grades: I, II, and III (5), or mild, moderate, and severe (1, 3, 8, 9).

Although intestinal metaplasia may be considered a dysplastic lesion (see Chapter 13), its common occurrence in the general population has caused many investigators to place it in the same category as the normal gastric mucosa. The metaplastic glands become dysplastic when their component cells are sufficiently abnormal, as illustrated later.

Based on currently available information and the opinions of panel members after reviewing the test microslides, the following general statements may be made:

The potential for malignant change in a gastric lesion is proportional to the severity of the dysplastic changes of its component cells.

Carcinoma may develop in a severely dysplastic epithelium.

Severely dysplastic epithelium and carcinoma may be morphologically similar, and clear differentiation between them may be difficult or even impossible, particularly in a biopsy specimen.

Moderate and severe grades of dysplasia often coexist and cannot be sharply distinguished from each other. Therefore, they may be considered in one category.

Mild dysplasia is not precancerous. It becomes precancerous when it progresses to higher grades.

The reversibility of dysplasia to a lower grade or to normal is likely for low-grade dysplasia. The reversibility is less likely for high-grade dysplasia and is questionable for severe dysplasia.

In view of the above, the Pathology Panel of the ISGGC recognizes that:

Abnormalities of gastric epithelium fall into two categories: hyperplasia and dysplasia.

Dysplasia is a precancerous lesion and includes both moderate and severe grades of abnormality.

Proliferative lesions of a nonprecancerous nature are hyperplastic but not dysplastic. Hyperplasia may be simple or severe and atypical, depending on the degree of hyperplasia and whether or not atypical cells are present.

When carcinoma cannot be excluded from consideration in a severely dysplastic epithelium, a diagnosis of possible carcinoma may be rendered so as to stimulate immediate reexamination and careful follow-up to obtain a more definitive diagnosis.

PATHOLOGICAL FEATURES OF DYSPLASIA AND RELATED LESIONS

The basic pathological features of gastric dysplasia are cellular atypia, abnormal differentiation, and disorganized architecture (9). They apply to both metaplastic and nonmetaplastic epithelia. In the normal stomach, the surface and foveolae are lined by a continuous, single-cell layer of tall, mucus-secreting, columnar cells. The regenerating zone is at the neck where occasional mitosis may be seen. The metaplastic glands have two basic forms: the complete type and the incomplete type. In the complete form, they are lined by absorptive cells interspersed with goblet cells. In the incomplete form, they are lined by goblet cells and mucous cells resembling the foveolar cells. The proliferative region is at the base of the gland.

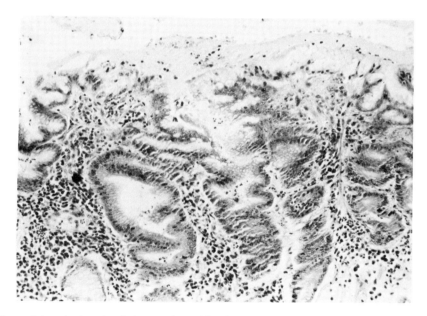

Figure 2-1.   Active simple hyperplasia. The foveolae are lined by an increased number of low columnar cells that mature and differentiate with increasing amounts of mucus secretion as they move toward the surface. There is intraglandular infolding, and the glands are dilated. This specimen was taken from an ulcer margin. H&E stain. × 150.

Simple Hyperplasia

There are two forms of simple hyperplasia (Figures 2-1 to 2-3). One is an active form and is seen at the site of active inflammation. This form is characterized by actively regenerating cells lining regular glandular tubules. The cells are columnar, uniform in size and shape, with basally located hyperchromatic nuclei, slightly basophilic cytoplasm, and occasional mitotic figures. The cells mature as they move to the surface, so that there is an increasing amount of mucus secretion in the surface cells.

When active simple hyperplasia involves a metaplastic mucosa, the lining cells of the glands are immature, goblet cells are few, and mucus secretion is low.

The other quiescent form of simple hyperplasia is seen in the hyperplastic polyp and Menetrier's disease and is characterized by inactive, mature cells lining irregular, usually dilated glands. The cells

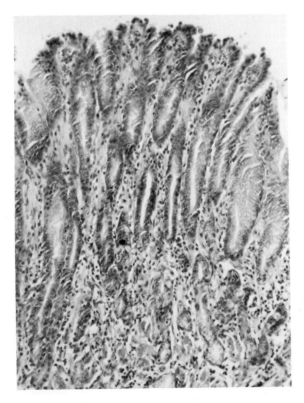

Figure 2-2.   Active simple hyperplasia. In this specimen the foveolae are lined by immature cells, with decreased mucus secretion all the way to the surface. The lower portions of the foveolae are lined by cuboidal cells. H&E stain. × 150.

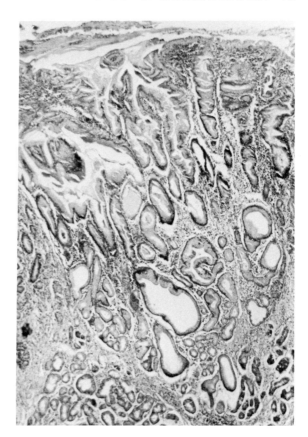

Figure 2-3.   Quiescent simple hyperplasia. There is an increased number of glands in the mucosa. These glands are dilated, and there are papillary infoldings of the lining cells, which are mature tall columnar cells with abundant mucus in the cytoplasm. This case had Menetrier's disease. H&E stain. × 60.

are well differentiated and tall columnar. Mitotic activity is generally absent.

Atypical or Severe Hyperplasia

Atypical hyperplasia (Figures 2-4 and 2-5) is an exaggerated form of active simple hyperplasia and is seen in various inflammatory conditions, eroded areas of hyperplastic polyps, occasional adenomas, mucosa adjacent to cancer, and the foveolar region of the mucosa in Menetrier's disease.

Compared with the epithelium in active simple hyperplasia, the cells in atypical hyperplasia are less uniform and more irregularly arranged. The immature cells extend all the way to the surface area. Mitotic figures are frequent. Intraluminal infolding and glandular branching are common.

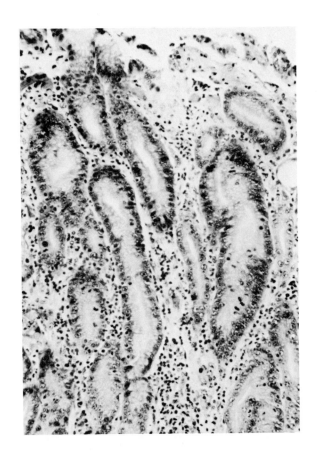

Figure 2-4. Atypical hyperplasia. The foveola are lined by immature cells with nucleoli and markedly decreased mucus secretion. There are many mitotic figures. H&E stain. ×150.

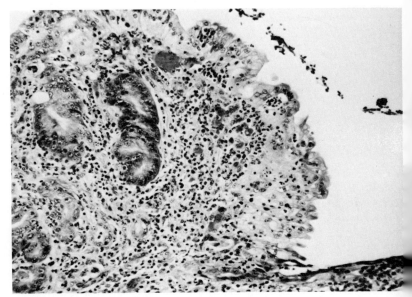

Figure 2-5. Atypical hyperplasia. The regenerated cells at the border of this chronic ulcer are pseudostratified. There is slight pleomorphism and loss of polarity. The glands at the left show active simple hyperplasia. H&E stain. ×150.

Dysplasia

Features of dysplasia (Figures 2-6 to 2-9) are characteristically shown by the adenomas. Dysplasia may be present in the mucosa adjacent to a carcinoma and in the stomach in various precancerous conditions. The degree of cellular abnormalities varies from moderate to severe. The cells are pleomorphic. Many cells have crowded, elongated nuclei. Others may have large, vesicular nuclei and prominent nucleoli. Pseudostratification is common and may be prominent. Mucus secretion is either scanty or more commonly absent. Intraluminal infolding may be present, usually mild, but budding and branching are prominent, resulting in the back-to-back arrangement of glands, particularly evident in the cross sections.

(Text continues on page 20)

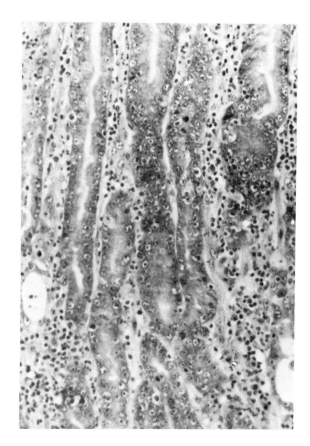

Figure 2-6. Dysplasia. The foveolae are lined by immature cells with prominent nucleoli and no mucus secretion. The cells are low columnar to cuboidal. The tubules are close to each other with a back-to-back arrangement. Some inflammatory cells have infiltrated the glands. H&E stain. × 200.

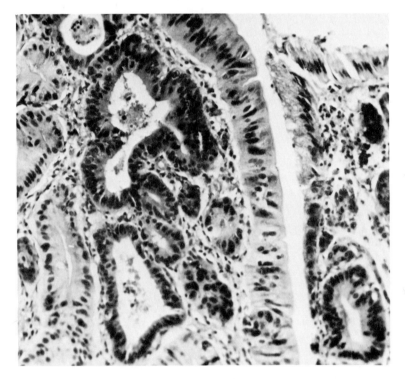

Figure 2-7.   Dysplasia of a metaplastic epithelium. The glands are lined by immature cells with hyperchromatism and pseudostratification. A striated border is clearly visible on the cells lining a long gland. There are no goblet cells. The glands along the left border are regular metaplastic glands without dysplasia. H&E stain. × 200.

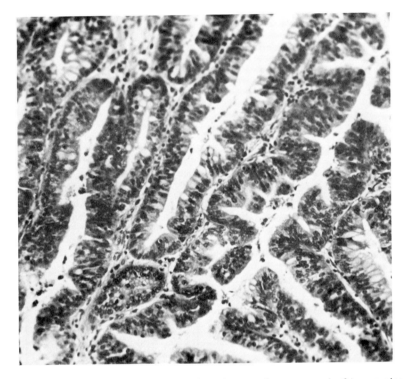

Figure 2-8.   Dysplasia of an adenoma. The adenoma is composed of incompletely metaplastic cells. The glands are lined by immature pseudostratified cells with prominent papillary infolding and branching. The mucous goblets are small. The intervening columnar cells have the appearance of foveolar cells with reduced mucus secretion. The nuclei of many cells are at the luminal surface. H&E stain. × 200.

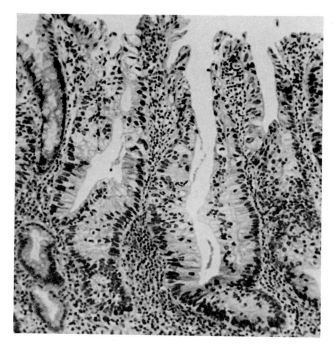

Figure 2-9.   Dysplasia. The glands are lined by pseudostratified cells with focal loss of polarity. A few cells have large nuclei. Most cells have reduced or no mucus secretion. The glands at left show metaplastic epithelium. H&E stain. × 150.

Possible Carcinoma

When the dysplastic changes are severe and cellular pleomorphism is prominent, it may be difficult to ascertain whether the dysplastic epithelium is still benign (i.e., dysplastic) or already malignant (i.e., carcinoma in situ). In the absence of clear evidence of microinvasion, a designation of possible carcinoma is appropriate (Figures 2-10 and 2-11).

The diagnosis of possible carcinoma is a temporary measure. Definitive diagnosis should be made as soon as possible by repeat biopsy.

Carcinoma In Situ, Microinvasive Carcinoma, and Intramucosal Carcinoma

Carcinoma in situ of the stomach is rarely observed as an isolated lesion. When the lesion is definitely malignant at the time of examination, microinvasion can usually be seen, if diligently searched for. If microinvasion is present, the lesion is malignant, even if the cellular

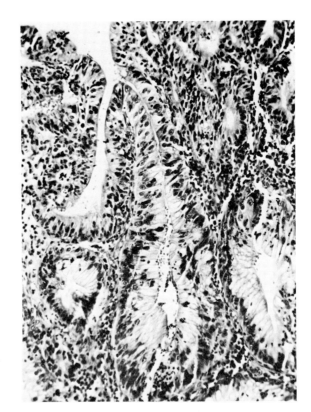

Figure 2-10. Possible cancer. The glands are lined by markedly dysplastic cells suggestive of malignancy. The final diagnosis was carcinoma when invasive cancer was found in the adjacent area. H&E stain. × 150.

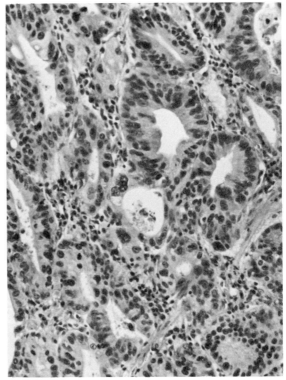

Figure 2-11. Possible cancer. The glandular epithelium at the center shows prominent pleomorphism with large nuclei. The glands are close together. However, most cells are uniform. Additional sections revealed no definite cancer, and the final diagnosis was adenoma with focal severe dysplasia. H&E stain. × 200.

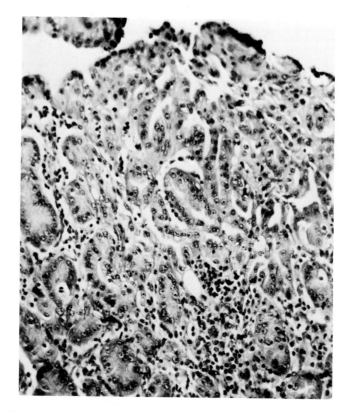

Figure 2-12.   Microinvasive carcinoma. The focus of the carcinoma is present in the superficial mucosa. The cells are poorly differentiated and cuboidal without mucus secretion. However, they are uniform and there is no mitosis. Their malignant nature is indicated by their arrangement. They form a solid mass with an ill-defined periphery, indicative of stromal invasion. The tubules at the left show active simple hyperplasia. H&E stain. × 150.

abnormalities are not severe (Figure 2-12). Without microinvasion, the diagnosis of carcinoma in situ must be made with great caution in order to avoid unnecessary gastrectomy.

Intramucosal carcinoma is an invasive carcinoma limited to the mucosa. Usually there is no difficulty in diagnosing it. Microinvasive carcinoma is an early intramucosal carcinoma, in that the invasion is focal and limited in extent so that it may be missed in the histological section or even in the biopsy specimen.

The pathological features of these lesions are summarized in Table 2-1 and their associated gastric diseases are listed in Table 2-2.

Table 2-1. Histological Features of Dysplasia and Related Lesions

Features	Simple Hyper-plasia	Atypical Hyper-plasia	Dys-plasia	Possible Cancer
Cellular abnormalities				
Immaturity and poor differentiation	1	2	3	3
No. of mitotic cells	1	2	1–3	1–3
Pseudostratification	0	1	0–3	0–3
Loss of polarity	0	0, 1	1, 2	1–3
Pleomorphism	0	0, 1	1, 2	2, 3
Anaplasia	0	0	1–3	2, 3
Abnormal mitotic figures	0	0	0, 1	0–2
Architectural derangements				
Elongation of glands	0–3	0–2	0–2	0–2
Dilatation of glands	0–3	0–2	0–2	0–2
Loss of normal deep glands	0–3	0–3	1–3	2, 3
Intraglandular folding	0–2	0–3	0–3	0–3
Budding and branching of glands	0–3	0–2	0–3	0–3
Crowding of glands	0	0–1	0–2	0–3
Back-to-back glands	0	0	0–2	0–3

0, absent; 1, slight; 2, moderate; 3, severe.
Note: The chief difference between cancer and possible cancer is the presence of stromal invasion in the former.

Table 2-2. Mucosal Changes in Various Benign Conditions

	Simple Hyperplasia	Atypical Hyperplasia	Dysplasia
Benign ulcer margin	+	±	±
Acute gastritis	+	−	−
Superficial chronic gastritis	+	−	−
Atrophic chronic gastritis	+	±	±
Gastric remnant	+	±	±
Menetrier's disease	+	±	±
Hyperplastic polyp	+	±	±
Adenoma	−	±	+
Mucosa bordering cancer	±	±	±

+ , usually present; − , usually absent; ± , occasionally present.

DISCUSSION

Most gastric cancer cells are poorly differentiated or anaplastic. Pleomorphism is prominent, and mitotic figures are often abnormal. Dysplastic cells are evaluated against this knowledge, and their potential for malignant change is graded according to the degree of abnormality. Thus, dysplasia has been graded from near normal to severely abnormal. It is generally accepted, however, that mild changes are probably not premalignant, since they are also found frequently in benign stomachs (5, 6). Furthermore, dysplasia may regress, even in the high grades (4). In view of these observations, the Pathology Panel of the ISGGC has advised the exclusion of mild abnormalities from the category of dysplasia in order to avoid unnecessary concern and over-zealous treatment. The classification system of the ISGGC is compared with other systems in Table 2-3.

Aside from the usual classification methods of grading the severity of abnormal changes, Cuello et al. (7) classified dysplasia into hyperplastic and adenomatous types, primarily for the metaplastic mucosa. Jass (9), using entirely different criteria, divided the dysplastic epithelium into two types: Type I epithelium, which resembled that of colonic adenoma and was found mainly in adenoma, and Type II epithelium, which was related to incomplete metaplasia and associated with poorly differentiated intestinal-type carcinoma.

Dysplastic epithelium has been shown to occur frequently in cancerous stomachs, particularly in association with the intestinal and expanding types of gastric cancer (6, 12). For these types of cancer, the

Table 2-3. Comparison of Different Grading Systems of Gastric Dysplasia

Nagayo (2)	No atypia	Slight atypia	Borderline	Probable cancer	Cancer
Grundmann and Schlake (3)	Inflammatory change	Mild	Moderate	Severe	
Oehlert et al. (5)	—	Grade I	Grade II	Grade III	
Ming (6)	Grade 1	Grade 2	Grade 3	Grade 4	
Cuello et al. (7)	Hyperplastic dysplasia mild	Hyperplastic dysplasia severe	Adenomatous dysplasia mild	Adenomatous dysplasia severe	
Morson et al. (1)	Inflammatory or regenerative change	Mild	Moderate	Severe	
ISGGC (1982)	Hyperplasia simple	Hyperplasia atypical	Dysplasia	Dysplasia possible carcinoma	

ISGGC, International Study Group on Gastric Carcinoma.

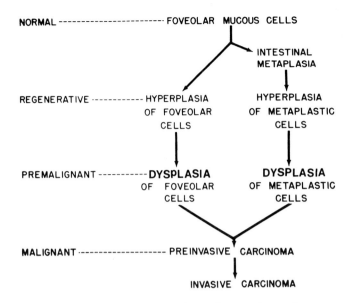

Figure 2-13.   Pathogenetic scheme for gastric carcinoma.

pathogenetic sequence shown in Figure 2-13 appears applicable. Similar observations have also been made in experimental carcinogenesis using N-methyl-N'-nitro-N-nitrosoguanidine as the carcinogen (17, 18). The diffuse and infiltrative types of gastric cancer, on the other hand, are not associated with any notable degrees of dysplasia, and their histogenetic processes remain unknown.

When dysplastic epithelium is found adjoining a cancer, it is generally accepted that the cancer has arisen from the dysplastic tissue. It is also possible, however, that the dysplasia and cancer are independent of each other even though they occur in the same stomach, as suggested by the finding of dysplastic epithelium away from the locus of gastric cancer (8). Furthermore, dysplasia, even of a high grade, has been found in many benign stomachs (5). Thus, dysplasia appears to be a nonspecific process that can be caused by several etiological factors and can occur in many different conditions, including carcinogenesis. The treatment of dysplasia, therefore, must be guided by its progression, which can be evaluated by follow-up studies.

Follow-up studies are necessary not only as a practical way of dealing with an individual case but also as an investigative measure to determine the frequency of malignant change. For the former the category of "possible carcinoma" is useful for facilitating the selection of cases that require immediate attention. Possible carcinoma includes, but is not limited to, the "borderline" lesion. To most pathologists a borderline lesion is a pathological ambiguity with cytological features in between malignancy and benignity so that a definite diagnosis is not possible. The term "borderline lesion" has also been applied by some to a specific elevated lesion that has also been called "atypical epithelium" (2, 19) and is most likely an adenoma (20). The term "possible carcinoma" applies to the former, not the latter, lesion.

Possible carcinoma may be a carcinoma already, but definite evidence of malignancy, such as stromal invasion, tumor giant cells, and bizarre mitotic figures, is lacking in the available biopsy specimen. It could be an in situ carcinoma (intraglandular carcinoma). Carcinoma in situ is a well-recognized clinical and pathological entity, particularly in the squamous epithelium. Theoretically it is a necessary stage of carcinogenesis, also applicable to the stomach. In practice, the intraglandular stage of gastric carcinoma without microinvasion is rarely observed, and its very existence as a diagnostic entity has been questioned (21). For those who recognize it, the presence of stromal invasion is required to support the diagnosis (22).

Possible carcinoma, therefore, is a temporary diagnosis and should be changed to a definitive diagnosis by repeat biopsy or biopsies so that proper therapy may be instituted without delay.

Since gastric dysplasia has been attracting a great deal of attention only recently, very few systematic investigations concerning it have been published. Further studies are needed to ascertain its natural history. Vital questions such as the frequency of dysplasia in various precancerous conditions and the frequency and latent duration of malignant change in a dysplastic epithelium can be answered by repeated endoscopic examinations. The classification system of abnormal gastric epithelium described in this chapter is offered to facilitate these studies.

REFERENCES

1. Morson, B. C., Sobin, L. H., Grundmann, E., Johansen, A., Nagayo, I., and Serck-Hanssen, A. Precancerous conditions and epithelial dysplasia in the stomach. *J. Clin. Pathol.* 33 (1980):711–721.
2. Nagayo, T. Histological diagnosis of biopsied gastric mucosae with special reference to that of borderline lesions. *Gann Monogr. Cancer Res.* 11 (1971):245–256.
3. Grundmann, E., and Schlake, W. Histology of possible precancerous stage in stomach. In *Gastric Cancer*, edited by Herfarth, Ch., and Schlag, P., pp. 72–82. Berlin: Springer-Verlag, 1979.

4. Oehlert, W. Biological significance of dysplasia of the epithelium and of atrophic gastritis. In *Gastric Cancer*, edited by Herfarth, Ch., and Schlag, P., pp. 91–104. Berlin: Springer-Verlag, 1979.

5. Oehlert, W., Keller, P., Henke, M., and Strauch, M. Gastric mucosal dysplasia: What is its clinical significance? *Front. Gastrointest. Res.* 4 (1979):173–182.

6. Ming, S.-C. Dysplasia of gastric epithelium. *Front. Gastrointest. Res.* 4 (1979):164–172.

7. Cuello, C., Correa, P., Zarama, G., Lopez, J., Murray, J., and Gordillo, G. Histopathology of gastric dysplasia. Correlations with gastric juice chemistry. *Am. J. Surg. Pathol.* 3 (1979):491–500.

8. Nagayo, T. Dysplasia of the gastric mucosa and its relation to the precancerous state. *Gann* 72 (1981):813–823.

9. Jass, J. R. A classification of gastric dysplasia. *Histopathology* 7 (1983):181–193.

10. Meister, H., Holubarsch, C. H., Haferkamp, O., Schlag, P., and Herfarth, Ch. Gastritis, intestinal metaplasia and dysplasia versus benign ulcer in stomach and duodenum and gastric carcinoma. A histotopographical study. *Pathol. Res. Pract.* 164 (1979):259–269.

11. Ming, S.-C., Goldman, H., and Freiman, D. G. Intestinal metaplasia and histogenesis of carcinoma in human stomach. Light and electron microscopic study. *Cancer* 20 (1967):1418–1429.

12. Grundmann, E. Histologic types and possible initial stages in early gastric carcinoma. *Beitr. Pathol.* 154 (1975):256–280.

13. Nagayo, T. Precursors of human gastric cancer: Their frequencies and histological characteristics. In *Pathophysiology of Carcinogenesis in Digestive Organs*, edited by Farber, E., pp. 151–161. Tokyo: University of Tokyo Press, 1977.

14. Siurala, M. Gastritis, its fate and sequelae. *Ann. Clin. Res.* 13 (1981):111–113.

15. Schrumpf, E., Serck-Hanssen, A., Stafaas, J., Aune, S., Myren, J., and Osnes, M. Mucosal changes in the gastric stump, 20–25 years after partial gastrectomy. *Lancet* 2 (1977):467–469.

16. Deschner, E. E., Winawer, S. J., and Lipkin, M. Patterns of nucleic acid and protein synthesis in normal human gastric mucosa and atrophic gastritis. *J. Natl. Cancer Inst.* 48 (1972):1567–1574.

17. Saito, T., Sasaki, O., Tamada, R., Iwamatsu, M., and Inokuchi, K. Sequential studies of development of gastric carcinoma in dogs induced by N-methyl-N'-nitro-N-nitrosoguanidine. *Cancer* 42 (1978):1246–1254.

18. Sigaran, M. F., and Con-Wong, R. Production of proliferative lesions in gastric mucosa of albino mice by oral administration of N-methyl-N'-nitro-N-nitrosoguanidine. *Gann* 70 (1979):343–352.

19. Sugano, H., Nakamura, K., and Takagi, K. An atypical epithelium of the stomach. A clinicopathological entity. *Gann Monogr. Cancer Res.* 11 (1971):257–269.

20. Oota, K. Early phase of development of human gastric cancer. *Gann Monogr. Cancer Res.* 18 (1976):77–83.

21. Kraus, B., and Cain, H. Is there a carcinoma in-situ of gastric mucosa? *Pathol. Res. Pract.* 164 (1979):342–355.

22. Schade, R. O. K. The borderline between benign and malignant lesions in the stomach. In *Early Gastric Cancer: Current Status of Diagnosis*, edited by Grundmann, E., Grunze, H., and Witte, S., pp. 45–53. Berlin: Springer-Verlag, 1974.

3 HISTOLOGICAL DIFFERENCES BETWEEN SEVERE DYSPLASIA AND PREINVASIVE CARCINOMA OF THE STOMACH

T. Nagayo

In the course of routine histological examination of resected stomachs, the author and other investigators (1–4) have found isolated, minute cancerous foci of less than 5 millimeters in diameter and have reported on their histological nature together with background findings. The foci were characterized by a clear-cut boundary to the surrounding mucosa, regardless of their histological nature. Some of them were microscopic in size. It is certain, therefore, that minute cancer represents an earliest stage in the development of gastric cancer.

It has also been noticed, however, that gastric cancers do not always start from such tiny focal lesions, but have a certain dimension from the very beginning. That is, there are not a few cases of widespread superficial mucosal changes showing the histology of adenocarcinoma nearly at the state of carcinoma in situ.

On the other hand, there are some lesions with borderline

change: Most of them are broad-based mucosal elevations, but some are depressed or deeply eroded. Both elevated and depressed lesions have some common histological features, that is, atypical epithelia of a foveolar nature in the upper half of the affected mucosa accompanied by nonatypical but cystically dilated glands in the lower half. There are not many cases of obvious adenocarcinoma within these borderline lesions, but the intermingling or coexistence of these two components in a single focus is not rare in the stomach.

For the study of the histogenesis of gastric cancer, therefore, it seemed necessary, or unavoidable, to introduce a concept of "dysplasia" in the field of gastric mucosa, as in the skin, uterine cervix, etc. This concept will contribute to the understanding of the nature of precancerous changes of the stomach.

DEFINITION AND CLASSIFICATION OF GASTRIC DYSPLASIA

The term "dysplasia" is defined as a lesion having the following three histological changes: cellular atypia; abnormal differentiation; and disorganized mucosal architecture. This idea was proposed by the World Health Organization's Subcommittee on Precancerous Changes of the Stomach in London in 1980 (5). Some authors (6–9) have already reported on this subject using this term. After slide seminars and discussions, the International Study Group on Gastric Cancer also adopted the term and the criteria for the changes related to precancerous lesions, even though some differences of opinion on its interpretation still exist among members.

The author has classified dysplasia into three grades—mild, moderate, and severe—and has reported on them previously (10, 11). The main purpose of the classification is to differentiate between nonmalignant and malignant change and between precancerous and cancerous change. From these viewpoints the histological criteria for severe dysplasia and the differences of the criteria from those for preinvasive cancer have utmost importance. These differences will be emphasized in this chapter.

DIFFERENCES IN HISTOLOGY BETWEEN SEVERE DYSPLASIA AND PREINVASIVE CARCINOMA

Even at the stage of intramucosal location, most cancers show invasive, infiltrative, or destructive growth regardless of their histological types, and no question would occur regarding the diagnosis of these

Table 3-1. Differences in Histology between Severe Dysplasia
and Preinvasive Carcinoma

	Severe Dysplasia	Preinvasive Carcinoma
From the aspect of component nuclei		
Pleomorphism	Not seen	Often seen
Nuclear-cytoplasmic ratio	Increased	Increased
Shape of nuclei	Relatively uniform	Varied
Stainability of nuclei	Mostly hyperchromatic	Varied
Arrangement of nuclei	Regular (dense and piled up)	Irregular (often dispersed)
From the aspect of cell differentiation		
Secretory granules	Decreased	Varied
Goblet and Paneth cells[a]	Decreased	Lost or increased
Distribution of mitotic cells	Less random	Random
Polarity of mitotic cells	Still maintained	Disturbed
Abnormal mitosis	Not seen	May be seen
From the aspect of glandular structure		
Form of tubules or glands	Still organized	Disorganized (as cordlike structure)
Running direction of tubules	Slightly disoriented	Markedly disoriented
Back-to-back fusion	Not seen	Often seen
Budding of small glands	Not seen	Often seen
Cystic dilatation of deeper glands	Quite often	Less often
Deformity of the cystic glands	Almost always	Not always

[a]Seen only in intestinal metaplasia.

cases. But when the cancer has a histological feature near the state of carcinoma in situ or in incipient phases, it is not easy for pathologists to diagnose it as definitely malignant. Differential diagnoses between incipient cancer and severe dysplasia are made chiefly from the experience of the examiner. Differential diagnoses should be as objective as possible; they are summarized in Table 3-1.

Regarding the cellular aspects, the features of the nuclei are essential. In general, the nuclear-cytoplasmic ratio is increased to a greater degree in carcinoma than in dysplasia, except for cases of the signet-ring cell series, in which the ratio is decreased to a greater extent in mature cancer cells than in normal counterparts owing to the accumulation of mucus in their cytoplasm. The shape of the nuclei is in general slender and monotonous in the lesion of dysplasia, whereas it is often oval or round with pleomorphism in that of tubular adenocarcinoma. Disarrangement of the nuclei is seen in both lesions, but is more marked in the cancerous epithelia than in the dysplastic ones. A piled-up arrangement of the hyperchromatic, elongated, but relatively uniform nuclei in tall columnar epithelia of a foveolar nature is characteristic of dysplasia, and such a change is usually not seen in obvious adenocarcinoma (Figures 3-1 to 3-3).

Abnormal differentiation of epithelia is recognizable by the loss of cytoplasmic secretory granules in cases of gastric-type lesions and

(Text continues on page 35)

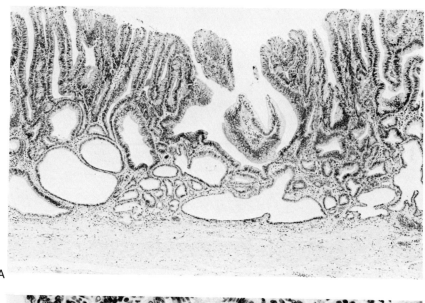

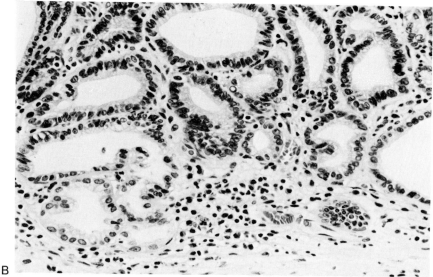

Figure 3-1.   Moderate dysplasia. The upper half of the slightly elevated mucosa is composed of tall columnar epithelia with elongated, hyperchromatic, but relatively uniform nuclei; irregularly dilated glands are seen in the lower half. The arrangement of the nuclei is well preserved in both components, and malignancy is not visible. H&E stain. × 40 (A); × 100 (B).

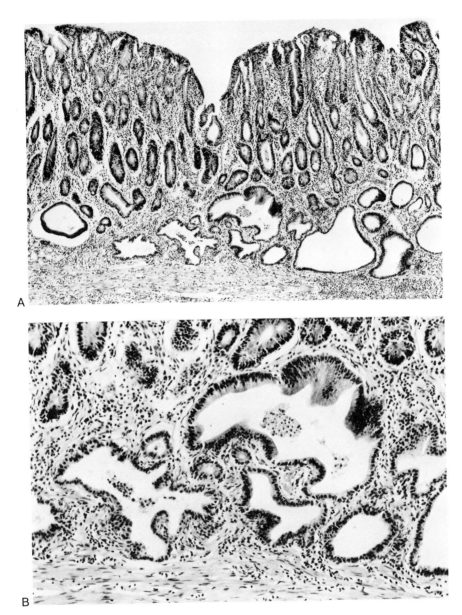

Figure 3-2. Severe dysplasia. Cellular atypia and structural abnormality are more intense than in the case shown in Figure 3-1. Irregularly dilated glands in the base of the lesion are composed of small cuboidal epithelia with a high nuclear-cytoplasmic ratio, but invasive growth suggesting malignancy is not seen. H&E stain. ×40 (A); ×100 (B).

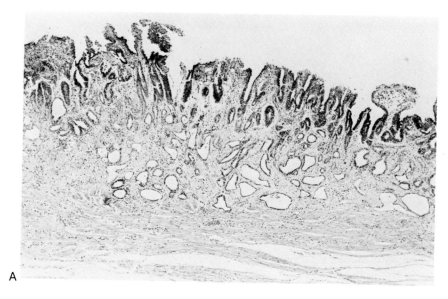

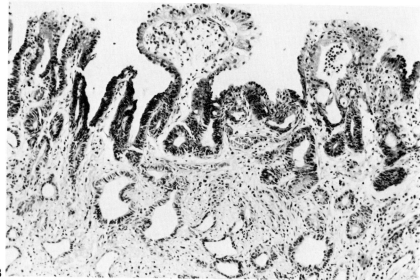

Figure 3-3.   Severe dysplasia. Regenerative mucosa following erosion shows typical dysplastic change. Irregularly dilated glands in the lower half of the mucosa are quite atypical from both cellular and structural aspects. Hyperchromatic tubules in the upper half also show some deformity, especially on the right. The incipient stage of cancer is quite doubtful, and no actual evidence of malignancy is seen. H&E stain. × 40 (**A**); × 100 (**B**).

the loss of goblet and Paneth cells in cases of metaplastic intestinal-type lesions. The loss is complete in cancer, whereas it is often incomplete in dysplasia. The distribution of mitotic cells is more random in cancer than in dysplasia, and the direction of the mitosis is also irregular in the former. Abnormal mitotic cells, which are not infrequently seen in cases of cancer, are hardly seen in cases of dysplasia.

The histological structures of the tubules and glands are more or less deformed in both lesions, but the loss of polarity as indicated by irregular branching or oblique running of the atypical tubules is more marked in cancer than in dysplasia. The budding of small glands composed of cuboidal epithelia lacking prominent cellular atypia but forming a cribriform structure, an irregular glandular network, and anastomosis of the neighboring tubular glands showing an X- or Y-shaped pattern are indicators of malignancy (Figures 3-4 and 3-5).

The replacement growth of atypical epithelia to neighboring nonatypical ones is seen in both types of lesions; therefore, this finding itself cannot be a characteristic of malignancy. Glandular cysts in the middle or lower layer of the affected mucosa are more frequently seen in dysplastic changes than in established cancer. Most of the cysts are composed of nonatypical but cuboidal cells. Irregularities in the form of dilated glands seen in the deeper layer are in general parallel to grades of cellular atypia of the foveolar tubules in cases of dysplasia, but this is not found in carcinoma.

SEVERE DYSPLASIA AND PRECANCEROUS CHANGE

Severe dysplasia is a histological concept and term, synonymous with precancerous change in its narrow sense. From the findings described above, it is certain that severe dysplasia is a proliferative, irreversible change and is destined to become cancer, sooner or later. There are several types of severe dysplasia, as shown in the figures, and it can be classified into two main types—gastric and intestinal—as in cancer. Several investigators (12–15) have described precancerous change of the stomach, and the histological changes presented in this volume can be interpreted with the criteria and grades of dysplasia set forth in this chapter.

CLINICAL IMPLICATION OF DYSPLASTIC CHANGES

Pathologists have a high possibility of encountering dysplastic changes in biopsied specimens. In that case histological diagnosis is of

(Text continues on page 38)

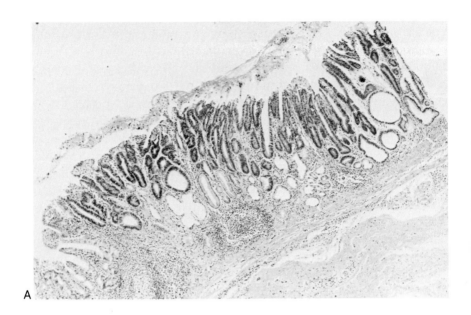

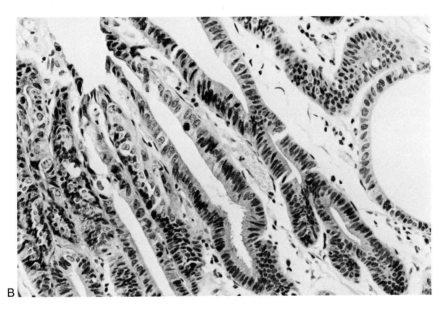

Figure 3-4.   Preinvasive adenocarcinoma. The upper half of the mucosa is diffusely occupied by hyperchromatic tubules composed mostly of tall columnar cells with well-arranged, rod-shaped, and hyperchromatic nuclei, but cuboidal cells with non-hyperchromatic, oval nuclei are interspersed among them. Structural abnormality is intense in this area. Mitotic cells are frequent, and their distribution is random. H&E stain. × 40 (**A**); × 200 (**B**).

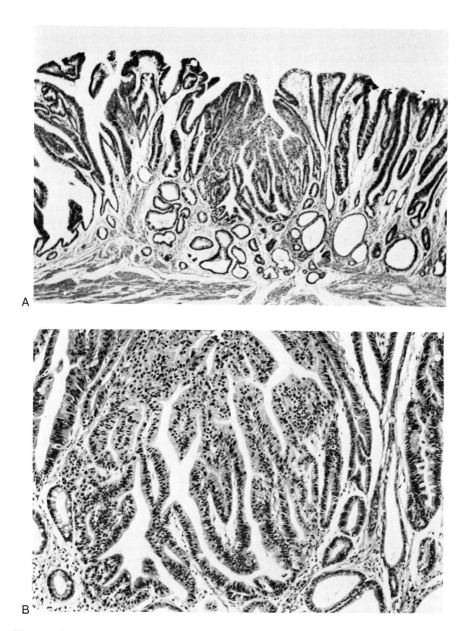

Figure 3-5.   Severe dysplasia coexisting with adenocarcinoma. The elevated mucosa essentially takes a form similar to that of villous adenoma. In this severely dysplastic mucosa, a tiny nodule composed of cuboidal and columnar epithelia forming papillary growth is visible. The arrangement of the small, spindle-shaped nuclei is already dispersed. These findings indicate that the papillary adenocarcinoma developed from the severely dysplastic lesion. H&E stain. × 40 (**A**); × 100 (**B**).

the utmost importance for patients and clinicians. In the author's opinion, when the changes seem to be in the state of severe dysplasia, a careful follow-up after a short interval (1 to 3 months) or an instant reexamination with biopsy, if possible, should be performed. In any case, the results of histological examination of the biopsy have to be compared with the findings obtained by radiographic and endoscopic examinations and analyzed carefully from various aspects before treatment is decided on.

SUMMARY

Differences of histology between severe dysplasia and preinvasive carcinoma of the stomach have been described from the aspects of cellular atypia, abnormal differentiation, and structural abnormality. Examples of both lesions were illustrated, and the histogenesis of gastric cancer was discussed.

REFERENCES

1. Nagayo, T. Microscopical cancer of the stomach—A study on histogenesis of gastric carcinoma. *Int. J. Cancer* 16 (1975):52–60.
2. Nakamura, K., Sugano, H., and Takagi, K. Histogenesis of carcinoma of the stomach less than 5mm in greatest diameter. Proceedings *10th International Cancer Congress, Houston,* 1970, p. 613.
3. Nakamura, K., Sugano, H., and Takagi, K. Carcinoma of the stomach in incipient phase. Its histogenesis and histological appearance. *Gann* 59 (1968):251–258.
4. Oohara, T., Tohma, H., Takezoe, K., Ukawa, S., Johjima, Y., Asakura, K., Aono, G., and Kurosawa, H. Minute gastric cancers less than 5mm in diameter. *Cancer* 50 (1982):801–810.
5. Morson, B. C., Sobin, S. H., Grundmann, E., Johansen, A., Nagayo, T., and Serck-Hanssen, A. Precancerous conditions and epithelial dysplasia in the stomach. *J. Clin. Pathol.* 33 (1980):711–721.
6. Oehlert, W., Keller, P., Henke, M., and Strauch, M. Die Dysplasien der Magenschleimhaut. Das Problem ihrer Klinischen Bedeutung. *Dtsch. Med. Wochenschr.* 100 (1975):1950–1956.
7. Oehlert, W. Gastric mucosal dysplasia: What is its clinical significance? *Front. Gastrointest. Res.* 4 (1979):173–182.
8. Ming, S.-C. Dysplasia of gastric epithelium. *Front. Gastrointest. Res.* 4 (1979): 164–172.
9. Cuello, C., Correa, P., Zarama, G., Lopez, J., Murray, J., and Gordillo, G. Histopathology of gastric dysplasia. Correlation with gastric juice chemistry. *Am. J. Surg. Pathol.* 3 (1979):491–500.
10. Nagayo, Y. Dysplastic changes of the digestive tract related to cancer. *Acta Endosc.* 10 (1980):69–80.

11. Nagayo, T. Dysplasia of the gastric mucosa and its relation to the precancerous state. *Gann* 72 (1981):813–823.
12. Serck-Hanssen, A. Precancerous lesions of the stomach. *Scand. J. Gastroenterol.* 54 (Suppl) (1979):164–165.
13. Correa, P. Precursors of gastric and esophageal cancer. *Cancer* 50 (1982): 2554–2565.
14. Grundmann, E. Histologic types and possible initial stages in the early gastric carcinoma. *Beitr. Pathol.* 154 (1975):256–280.
15. Grundmann, E. Classification and clinical consequences of precancerous lesions in the digestive and respiratory tracts. *Acta Pathol. Jpn.* 33 (1983):195–217.

4 EPITHELIAL DYSPLASIA OF THE STOMACH AND ITS RELATIONSHIP WITH GASTRIC CANCER

Y. Zhang

As a pathologic entity, epithelial dysplasia of the gastric mucosa has attracted special attention in the study of gastric carcinoma. Many pathologists have accepted that epithelial dysplasia of the gastric mucosa is a precancerous lesion (1–11). However, there is confusion about its typing and grading (1–3, 6, 10). Since the behavior of epithelial dysplasia and the relationship between dysplasia and gastric carcinoma are not yet clear, we collected the following materials hoping to find some information that would clarify the problems stated above.

MATERIALS AND METHODS

The materials consisted of 101 specimens accumulated during the last 20 years. They included: 41 cancerous stomachs with epithelial dysplasia from among 572 cases of gastric carcinoma resected surgically from 1960 to 1980; 18 nonmalignant stomachs with epithelial dysplasia from among 67 cases resected surgically during the same period; and 42 mucosal biopsy specimens with epithelial dysplasia from among 3,272 cases.

The resected stomachs were all dissected along the great curvature; they were then spread out, pinned onto a wax board, and fixed in 10% formalin after thorough gross examination. In advanced carcinoma, about ten blocks were taken, whereas in most early carcinoma specimens, serial blocks of the whole carcinoma and its adjacent mucosa within 1 to 2 centimeters were cut for sectioning. In a few cases the whole stomach was cut serially. The mucosal biopsies were divided into two groups, the antrum and the body groups, and serial sections were made. Hematoxylin and eosin (H&E) stain was routinely applied. In addition, alcian blue (pH 2.5)/periodic acid-Schiff (AB/PAS), alcian blue (pH 1.0), periodic acid-borohydride/potassium hydroxide/periodic acid-Schiff (PB/KOH/PAS) (12), and high-iron diamine/alcian blue (pH 2.5) (HID/AB) (13) stains were used in many cases to show the characteristics of mucin.

RESULTS

Gross Appearance of Epithelial Dysplasia in the Surgically Resected Specimens

The majority of the dysplastic lesions in the surgically resected specimens were discovered upon microscopic examination. Only a few cases were found upon gross examination because they were somewhat excavated or eroded. Some cases showed abnormalities of color and luster (gray-yellow or gray-red). The dysplastic foci in these cases were microscopic. Occasionally, the dysplastic lesion involved a relatively large area (about 1 centimeter in diameter).

In nine cases the dysplastic lesion exhibited a semispherical shape or a flat, elevated patch, just like the early gastric carcinomas of IIa or IIa + IIc types, and measured less than 1.0 centimeter. The outline of these foci was relatively clear-cut, and the surface was rough, especially in the slightly depressed central portion. These dysplastic foci were called flat adenomas by many pathologists. Seven cases had a single focus, and five of these had accompanying gastric carcinoma in the adjacent area (Figure 4-1). The dysplastic foci were located in the antrum in seven and the transition zone in two cases.

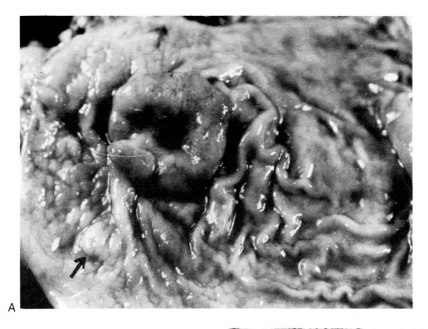

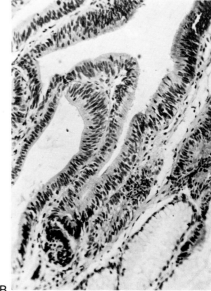

Figure 4-1.   Gross specimen of a
stomach with flat adenoma (adenomatous dysplasia) near a fungating-type gastric carcinoma (A). The histopathologic
appearance of the dysplastic lesion
shows an adenoma with severe-grade
epithelial dysplasia (B). H&E stain.
×210.

Histopathological Appearance of Epithelial Dysplasia

The main histopathological and cytological features of epithelial dysplasia were disorganized architecture of the glands and abnormal dif-

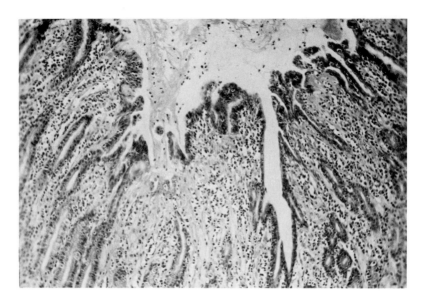

Figure 4-2.   Mild dysplasia in an erosion in gastritis verrucosa. H&E stain. × 120.

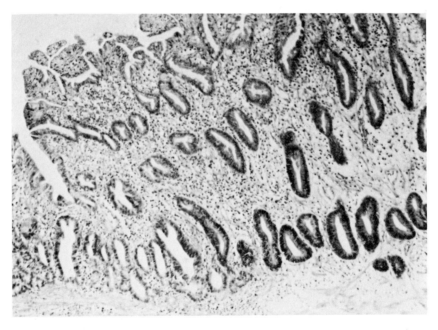

Figure 4-3.   Dysplasia of intestinal metaplastic mucosa in atrophic gastritis. In the deep portion of the atrophied mucosa, note the mild dysplastic lesions on the right side, and many glands suspected of malignancy on the left. H&E stain. × 120.

ferentiation of the cells. The involved epithelium might be of the gastric type or the intestinal metaplastic type.

Three grades of severity could be identified.

Mild Grade (39 Cases) In the mild grade the dysplastic epithelium sometimes exhibited disorganization of the glands only, and the cellular atypism and secreting function of the epithelial cells were only slightly affected. In the gastric epithelium, the mucous material was slightly diminished or well maintained. Mild dysplasia could be found mainly in the margin of ulcers or erosions (Figure 4-2). In the intestinalized epithelium, there was a diminishing or absence of globlet cells, usually at the deep portion of the metaplastic glands (Figure 4-3).

The disorganized glands were arranged in two fashions: In some cases, the glands were tortuous and packed together closely (Figure 4-4); in other cases, the dysplastic glands were widely separated (Figure 4-2).

The demarcation between the dysplastic focus and adjacent normal glands was not clear-cut. Transitional features between the ordinary intestinal metaplasia and dysplasia could usually be seen. It is believed that this is the early stage of epithelial dysplasia, although early cancerization was found among these dysplastic glands in one case.

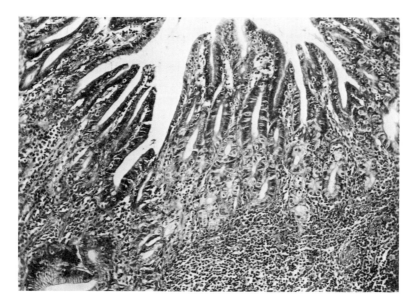

Figure 4-4.   Mild dysplasia in an eroded focus of the gastric mucosa. Tubules are arranged closely. H&E stain. × 120.

Moderate Grade (15 Cases) In the moderate grade both irregularity of the glandular architecture and atypia of the epithelium were more distinct than in mild dysplasia. The lumina of glands were not uniform and were generally wider than normal. Budding and/or branching and occasionally back-to-back arrangement of the glands could be seen (Figure 4-1B). The dysplastic glands were often packed closely. This grade of dysplasia was usually seen in flat adenoma.

The cytoplasm of dysplastic cells with brush borders was relatively deeply stained with H&E stain (Figure 4-1B). The nuclei had an elongated shape and were rich in chromatin. Typical goblet and Paneth cells were often absent. The cellular arrangement was irregular and pseudostratified (Figures 4-1B and 4-5). Occasional mitotic figures were present.

Severe Grade (47 Cases) In the severe grade many foci were located in the vicinity of carcinoma (mostly early carcinoma); some were distinct from its outline and some were not (Figure 4-6). Atypia of the cells was characterized by nuclear pleomorphism. Some cells were columnar, but they were usually cuboid or irregularly shaped

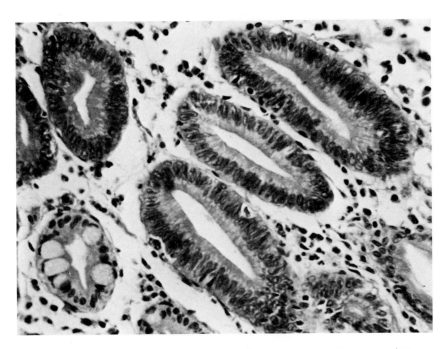

Figure 4-5.   Moderate dysplasia of absorptive-type cells. H&E stain. ×410.

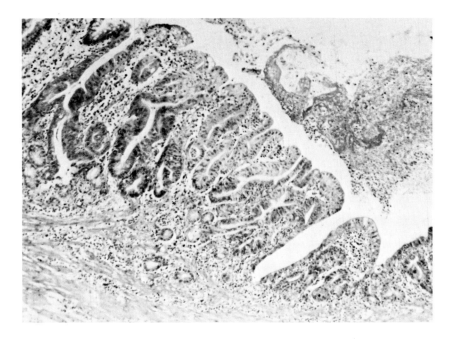

Figure 4-6.   Severe epithelial dysplasia (**left**) without clear-cut demarcation from the carcinomatous focus (**right**). The dysplastic cells show hyperchromasia and pleomorphism. H&E stain. × 120.

(Figure 4-6). The nuclear-cytoplasmic ratio was obviously increased. The nuclei were rich in chromatin and not uniform. Mitotic figures were sometimes seen. The severely dysplastic epithelium sometimes could not be distinguished from the highly differentiated microcarcinoma. In this case suspected carcinoma was diagnosed.

Histochemistry of the Dysplastic Epithelium

When stained with HID/AB, regardless of the grade of dysplasia, the intestinalized cells were shown to have only a trace of sialomucin and various amounts of sulfomucin at their free surface (Figure 4-7). As a whole the amount of sulfomucin was markedly increased in the dysplastic epithelia. Sometimes, many clumps of it appeared in the apical pole of severely dysplastic epithelia and epithelia suspected of malignancy (Figure 4-8). Almost no O-acetyl sialomucin could be detected in dysplastic epithelia with PB/KOH/PAS stain. In mild dysplasia of gastric-type epithelium, only neutral mucin or a trace amount of sialomucin could be seen.

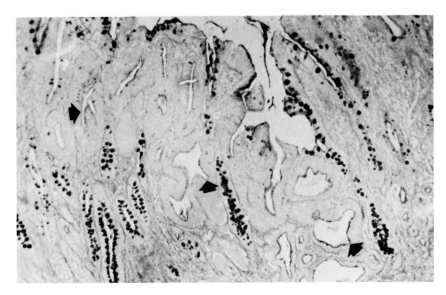

Figure 4-7.   Dysplastic epithelium in an adenoma stained with HID/AB. The goblet cells in the intestinalized gland at the border of dysplastic lesion are stained blue (shown as black), indicating the presence of sialomucin; the dysplastic epithelia are unstained, but the brush borders (*arrows*) are stained brown-black (shown as gray), indicating the presence of sulfomucin. × 120.

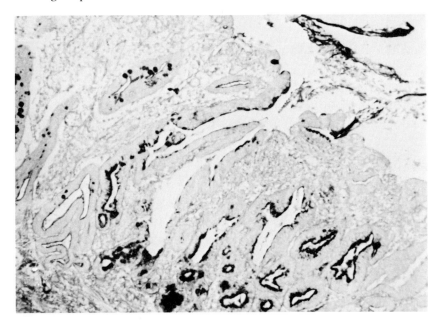

Figure 4-8.   The same lesion as shown in Figure 4-6 stained with HID/AB. The cancer cells contain sulfomucin (black clumps and granules) in their apical portions (**right**). In the dysplastic epithelia, many cells have the same appearance as the cancer cells, whereas others are stained brown-black on brush borders only (**left**). × 120.

Pathologic Changes of the Gastric Mucosa Surrounding the Dysplastic Lesion

In 42 mucosal biopsy specimens, dysplasia involved intestinalized epithelium in 21 and gastric epithelium in 21. Severe intestinal metaplasia was present in the surrounding mucosa in 11 (52.3 percent) of the former and 3 (14.3 percent) of the latter cases. In nine cases of flat adenoma, atrophic gastritis with intestinal metaplasia was seen in its adjacent mucosa (antrum) in eight (88.9 percent). The remaining case had superficial gastritis with mild intestinal metaplasia. All carcinomas accompanying dysplasia were highly differentiated papillotubular adenocarcinomas, i.e., intestinal-type carcinomas. These findings demonstrate that there is a definite relationship between the histologic type of epithelium in dysplasia and the histopathologic type of gastric carcinoma.

Malignant Alteration of Epithelial Dysplasia

Two approaches were available for the study of the malignant alteration of epithelial dysplasia. One was to find the topographic relationship and transitional features between epithelial dysplasia and carcinoma in the same specimen; the other was the follow-up study of the dysplastic lesion. These approaches are described.

Topographic Distribution and Transitional Features In 41 cases dysplastic epithelium was found in cancerous stomachs (16 cases of early carcinoma and 25 cases of advanced carcinoma). Many dysplastic foci were found to be in continuation with the carcinoma. It was not certain, however, whether they developed independently or the dysplastic lesions preceded the carcinomas.

Follow-Up Study Carcinoma developed in three cases of epithelial dysplasia during the follow-up period. Two of these cases were found in a mass survey. One and one-half years later, they were proved to have early gastric carcinoma by endoscopic biopsy examination. The other case was an outpatient, and gastric dysplasia was discovered by endoscopic biopsy. Two years later at reexamination, the dysplastic lesion could not be determined to be either benign or malignant. The stomach was resected and an early gastric carcinoma measuring 1.5 centimeters was found.

Multiple Gastric Carcinoma and Epithelial Dysplasia

Among 572 cancerous stomachs collected from 1960 to 1980, we found 26 cases of multiple gastric carcinomas. In 11 of them the carcinoma was accompanied by epithelial dysplasia (42.3 percent),

Table 4-1. Multiple Gastric Carcinoma and Epithelial Dysplasia

Groups of Carcinoma	No. of Specimens	Dysplasia	
		No.	%
Single focus	546	30	5.5
Multiple foci	26	11	42.3

whereas only 30 cases of dysplasia were found in 546 cases of single gastric carcinoma (Table 4-1).

Incidence of Epithelial Dysplasia in Early and Advanced Gastric Cancers

It was noted that epithelial dysplasia was more common in stomachs with early carcinoma than in advanced cases (Table 4-2).

DISCUSSION

Epithelial dysplasia of the gastric mucosa is the result of a deviation of differentiation from normal epithelial cells. The morphological characteristics of dysplasia consist mainly of disorganization of the architecture of glands and dedifferentiation and atypia of the affected epithelial cells. The degree of epithelial dysplasia denotes the degree of dedifferentiation and abnormal biological behavior of the epithelial cells. Dysplasia has been divided into many grades (1, 4–6, 9). In this chapter three grades of dysplastic lesions were given, i.e., mild, moderate, and severe, or suspected of malignancy. The last also conveys a state of borderline changes; i.e., the benignity or malignancy of the lesion cannot be determined. It is felt that in these cases, many lesions may already have the character of malignancy. At the other end of the spectrum, we think it is better to avoid the diagnosis of dysplasia for the mild grade as it has no clinical significance.

Table 4-2. Incidence of Epithelial Dysplasia Found in Early and Advanced Gastric Cancers

Groups of Carcinoma	Case No.	Dysplasia	
		No.	%
Early carcinoma	41	16	39.0
Advanced carcinoma	531	25	4.7

In the search for other indexes to denote the difference between benign and malignant dysplastic lesions, we examined the mucous materials contained in the epithelial cells. Acid mucins, particularly the sulfomucins, detected by HID/AB stain may be helpful in this regard. As we know from the histochemical studies of intestinal metaplasia and gastric cancer, a metaplastic epithelium secreting sulfomucin may be of a precancerous nature, especially in adenomatous polyps with dysplastic epithelia.

The relationship between epithelial dysplasia and gastric cancer and the incidence rate of malignant transformation from dysplasia have until now not been clear. According to this study, the precancerous nature or malignant potential of dysplasia is certain, although the duration required for malignant transformation is still unknown. As mentioned above, epithelial dysplasias were more common in stomachs bearing early cancer than in advanced cases (Table 4-2). This indicates that the dysplastic lesions may have developed before the carcinoma occurred. If dysplasia was a secondary change, we should have found more dysplasia in the stomachs with advanced cancer. Follow-up studies also confirmed the precancerous nature of dysplasia, but more cases and detailed observations are needed.

SUMMARY

Epithelial dysplasia in 59 cases of surgically resected stomach and 42 cases of mucosal biopsy specimens was reported. Descriptions of the macroscopic and microscopic characteristics and its gradings were given. According to the degree of disorganization of the glandular architecture and dedifferentiation and atypia of the gastric epithelial cells, dysplasia was divided into three grades: mild, moderate, and severe. The relationship between epithelial dysplasia and carcinoma was discussed. It is believed that epithelial dysplasia is an important precancerous lesion of the stomach. The precancerous nature of dysplasia was indicated by its high incidence in cancerous stomachs, particularly in those with early carcinoma, and by the development of early cancer in three cases of dysplasia during the follow-up period.

REFERENCES

1. Nagayo, T. Borderline lesion of gastric mucosa—Elevated and excavated type [English summary]. *Stomach Intest.* 10 (1975):1437–1442.

2. Hakamura, K. Histological study on early carcinoma of the stomach: Criteria for diagnosis of atypical epithelium. *Gann* 57 (1966):613–620.
3. Cuello, C., Correa, G., Lopez, J., and Gordillo, G. Histopathology of gastric dysplasia. Correlations with gastric juice chemistry. *Am. J. Surg. Pathol.* 3 (1979):491–500.
4. Cuello, C., and Correa, P. Dysplastic changes of the gastric mucosa. In *Gastric Cancer*, edited by Herfarth, Ch., and Schlag, P., pp. 83–90. Berlin: Springer-Verlag, 1979.
5. Grundmann, E., and Schlake, W. Histology of possible precancerous stages in the stomach. In *Gastric Cancer*, edited by Herfarth, Ch., and Schlag, P., pp. 72–82. Berlin: Springer-Verlag, 1979.
6. Ming, S.-C. Dysplasia of gastric epithelium. *Front. Gastrointest. Res.* 4 (1979): 164–172.
7. Oehlert, W. Biological significance of dysplasias of the epithelium and atrophic gastritis. In *Gastric Cancer*, edited by Herfarth, Ch. and Schlag, P., pp. 91–104. Berlin: Springer-Verlag, 1979.
8. Meister, H., Holubarsch, Ch., Haferkamp, O., Schlag, P., and Herfarth, Ch. Significance and location of atrophic gastritis and of glandular dysplasia in benign and malignant gastric disease. In *Gastric Cancer*, edited by Herfarth, Ch., and Schlag, P., pp. 105–107. Berlin: Springer-Verlag, 1979.
9. Zhang, Y. C., Bai, Y. Z., and Zhang, W. F. Histopathologic study of atypical epithelial proliferation of the gastric mucosa and its follow-up study. [English abstract]. *Chin. J. Oncol.* 1 (1979):23–28.
10. Morson, B. C., Sobin, L. H., Grundmann, E., Johansen, A., Nagayo, T., and Serck-Hanssen, A. Precancerous conditions and epithelial dysplasia in the stomach. *J. Clin. Pathol.* 33 (1980):711–721.
11. Sano, R. *Surgical Pathology of Gastric Diseases*, 3rd ed. [Japanese], pp. 224–233. Tokyo: Igaku Shoin Ltd., 1974.
12. Culling, C. E. A., Reid, P. E., Burton, J. D., and Dunn, W. L. A. A histochemical method of differentiating lower gastrointestinal tract mucin from other mucins in primary or metastatic tumors. *J. Clin. Pathol.* 28 (1975):656–658.
13. Spicer, S. S. Diamine methods for differentiating mucosubstances histochemically. *J. Histochem. Cytochem.* 13 (1965):211–234.

5 EPITHELIAL DYSPLASIA IN THE STOMACH: THE SIZE OF THE PROBLEM AND SOME PRELIMINARY RESULTS OF A FOLLOW-UP STUDY

A. Serck-Hanssen, M. Osnes, and J. Myren

The term "dysplasia," although originally implying a disturbance of development, is now also commonly used for histological and cytological changes believed to be precancerous. At least in Europe, the term is commonly used for organs covered by squamous epithelium, particularly the uterine cervix.

In the field of gastric pathology, however, histopathological changes believed to be precancerous have been given different names by different workers (1–12). This has caused some confusion among both clinicians and pathologists, and has to a certain extent retarded the general progress in understanding the natural behavior and hence the clinical significance of these lesions.

In an attempt to reach agreement on the histopathological criteria and nomenclature of precancerous changes in the stomach, a meeting was held in London, U.K., in 1978 on the initiative of B. C. Morson and supported by the World Health Organization (WHO), the Union Internationale Contre le Cancer, and the International Cancer Research Workshop Programme. The meeting was attended by six pathologists from different countries (B. C. Morson, England; L. H. Sobin, U.S.A. and WHO; E. Grundmann, F.R.G.; A. Johansen, Denmark; T. Nagayo, Japan; and A. Serck-Hanssen, Norway). The recommended criteria and nomenclature set forth by this group were published in 1980 (13). The main points related to dysplasia in the stomach were the following.

1. Mucosal changes believed to be precancerous should be called "dysplasia." Epithelial changes believed to be inflammatory should be called "regenerative" or "reactive" (Figures 5-1 and 5-6).

2. The main histological features of dysplasia are cellular atypia, abnormal differentiation, and disorganized mucosal architecture (Figures 5-2 to 5-5 and 5-7 to 5-11).

3. These dysplastic epithelial changes may be seen in the gastric surface or foveolar epithelium (Figures 5-2 to 5-5) as well as in the intestinal metaplastic epithelium (Figures 5-7 to 5-11), both of which may be the source of carcinoma (Figures 5-5C,D and 5-8B,C).

The degree of change varies from mild dysplasia (Figures 5-2 and 5-7), which must be separated from changes believed to be reactive or inflammatory (Figures 5-1 and 5-6), through moderate dysplasia (Figures 5-3, 5-5, and 5-8) to severe dysplasia (Figures 5-4, 5-10, and 5-11), which is a lesion reminiscent of carcinoma but in which clear evidence of invasion of the lamina propria is lacking. The use of the term "severe dysplasia" is recommended instead of "carcinoma in situ" to avoid confusion with "intramucosal carcinoma," which is a real invasive carcinoma but limited to the mucosa (Figures 5-4, 5-5, and 5-8C).

The recognition of dysplasia and an agreement on the criteria and grading of this lesion are felt to be important for several reasons:

1. A proper understanding of the natural history of gastric dysplasia and hence its significance can be achieved only if a sufficient number of patients are followed through a sufficient length of time in properly conducted prospective series in different parts of the world, by a number of pathologists who agree on its criteria and grading.

2. We believe that dysplasia is a histopathological sign that marks patients at risk for development of gastric cancer over and above that of patients with precancerous conditions, as defined by the WHO

(Text continues on page 63)

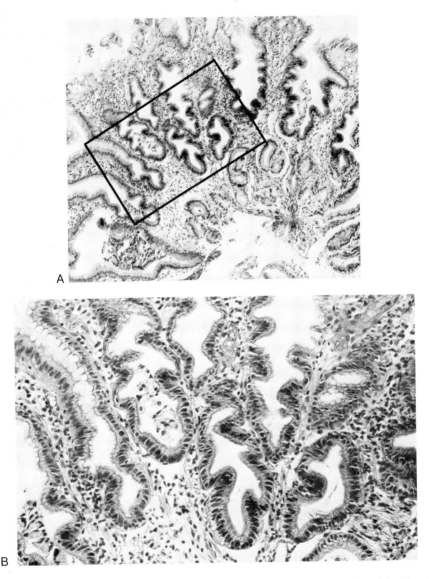

Figure 5-1.   Gastroscopic biopsy from antrum reveals marked atrophy with dilated foveolar crypt with small papillary structures. The foveolar epithelium is slightly more basophilic than normal. The marked area in (A) is shown in (B). In (B) is seen a slight nuclear pleomorphism and the absence or abnormal location of secretory vacuoles, i.e., between the nucleus and the basement membrane. The changes, however, are slight and considered within the range of an inflammatory, regenerative reaction. H&E stain. × 80 **(A)**; × 210 **(B)**.

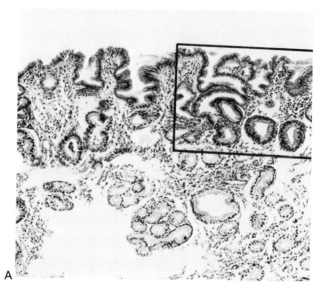

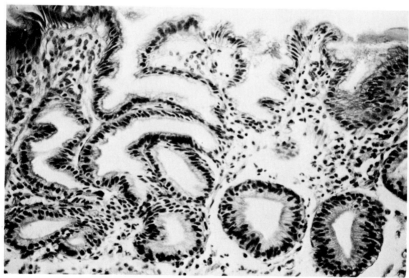

Figure 5-2.   Biopsy shows markedly atrophic antral mucosa with many of the same features illustrated in Figure 5-1. In addition is seen in the right half of the field a small area (marked) of disorganized mucosal architecture with back-to-back formation of foveolar crypts. Under greater magnification (B) crypts can be seen to be lined by slightly enlarged cells with mild nuclear pleomorphism and early nuclear stratification. Changes are considered to be mild dysplasia of the gastric type. H&E stain. × 80 (A); × 210 (B).

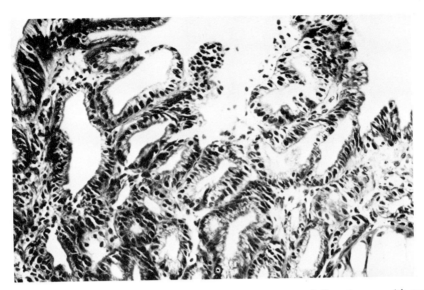

Figure 5-3.   Antral biopsy shows fairly marked architectural disturbance with surface papillary structures and adenomatous hyperplasia of foveolar structures with back-to-back formations. Nuclear pleomorphism is moderately marked. There is no evidence of intestinal metaplasia. Diagnosis was moderate dysplasia of the gastric type. H&E stain. × 210.

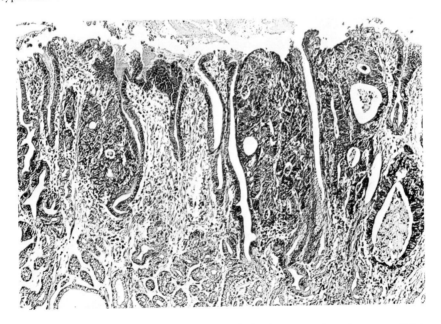

Figure 5-4.   Gastric remnant removed after Billroth II resection shows small intramucosal carcinoma in separate foci. The surface and foveolar epithelium show no evidence of intestinal metaplasia, but marked cellular atypia in gastric-type epithelium. This lesion is considered to demonstrate intramucosal carcinoma of gastric epithelial origin. H&E stain. × 80.

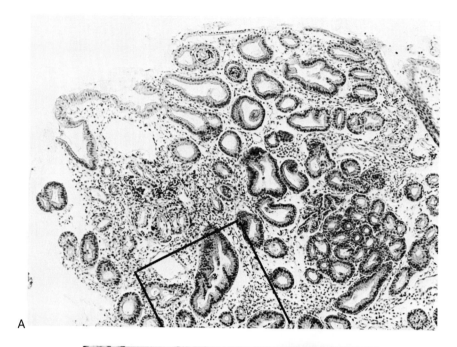

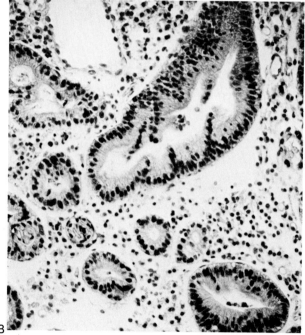

Figure 5-5 (Continues).

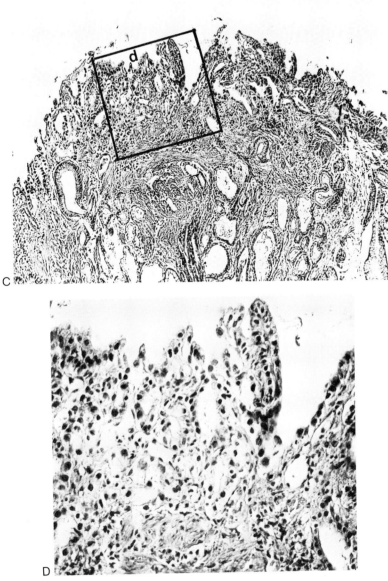

Figure 5-5. All parts from the same patient: a male, born in 1924, who underwent Billroth II resection in 1946 for duodenal ulcer. **A** and **B**: One of 20 gastroscopic biopsies taken in 1977, which shows a small area with irregular foveolar crypts with small intraluminal papillary structures (**window** in A) which reveal slight nuclear pleomorphism and stratification under higher magnification (B). This was diagnosed as moderate dysplasia of the gastric type. Annual follow-up with multiple biopsies from posterior gastric wall near efferent loop was carried out. **C** and **D**: One of two positive biopsies taken in May 1983, which shows a small area superficially in the mucosa (**window** in C). Under higher magnification (D) this area shows loss of normal foveolar structures, marked cellular atypia, enlarged hyperchromatic nuclei, and early invasion in the lamina propria. This was diagnosed as intramucosal carcinoma. H&E stain. ×80 (**A**); ×210 (**B, D**); ×35 (**C**).

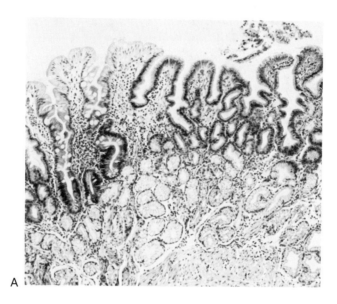

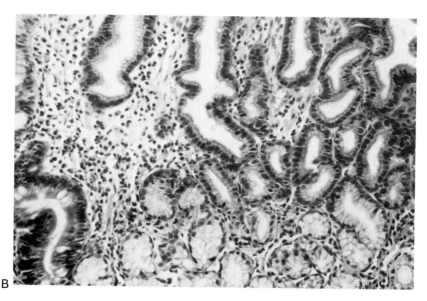

Figure 5-6.   Gastroscopic biopsy from antrum shows chronic, slightly atrophic gastritis with intestinal metaplasia in two foveolar crypts. Slight loss of differentiation is manifested by a reduced number of goblet cells toward the bottom of the crypts, with some elongation and stratification of nuclei. Note also slight changes in the gastric-type foveolar cells, with moderately enlarged nuclei but no pleomorphism. This was diagnosed as reactive inflammatory changes in both metaplastic intestinal and gastric foveolar epithelium. H&E stain. × 80 (A); × 210 (B).

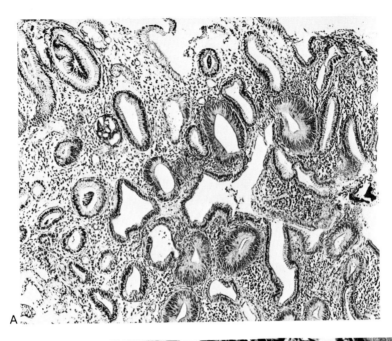

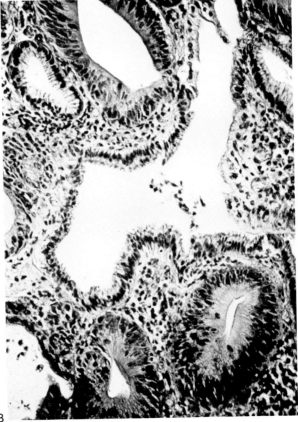

Figure 5-7. Gastroscopic biopsy from antrum shows disturbed mucosal architecture with several foveolar crypts in central field (**A**), lined by dedifferentiated intestinal epithelium (no goblet cells). Greater magnification (**B**) shows a distinct brush border and enlarged, stratified nuclei with mitoses in the lining cells of three of these crypts. This was diagnosed as mild dysplasia in an area of intestinal metaplasia. H&E stain. ×80 (**A**); ×230 (**B**).

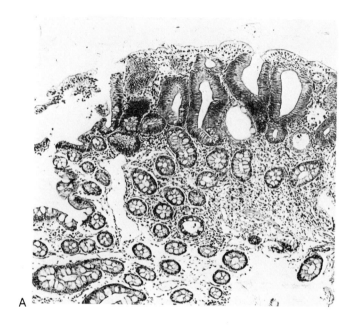

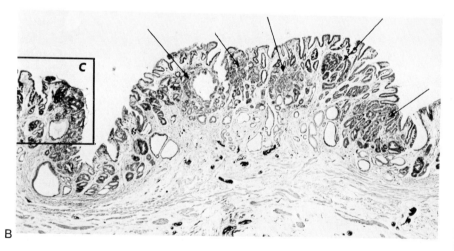

Figure 5-8 (Continues).

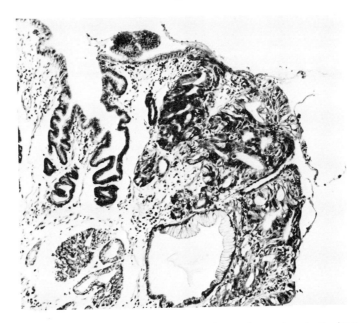

Figure 5-8   **A**: Gastroscopic biopsy from a small, elevated area close to the border of a peptic ulcer reveals four foveolar crypts lined by dedifferentiated and atypical cells of the intestinal type. Occasional remnants of small goblet cells, a distinct brush border, elongated hyperchromatic nuclei with stratification, and several mitoses are also seen. This was diagnosed as dysplastic intestinal metaplasia, atypia close to severe. Because of malignant cells in the brush cytology, a resection was done (B). **B**: Section through an elevated area shows several foci with dysplasia (*arrows*) and a small area with intramucosal carcinoma (**window**). **C**: Section shown in (B) under higher magnification. H&E stain. × 80 (**A**); × 30 (**B**); × 100 (**C**).

(14). For instance, chronic atrophic gastritis with intestinal metaplasia has long been recognized to be associated with an increased risk of developing gastric cancer (15–18). The number of patients within this group, however, is too large to be followed by regular gastroscopies with biopsies. In the Department of Pathology at Ullevål Hospital, Oslo, Norway, approximately 500 patients per year are found to have

(Text continues on page 66)

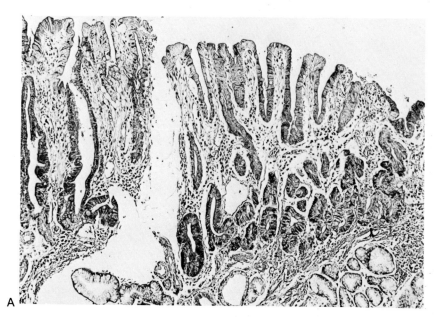

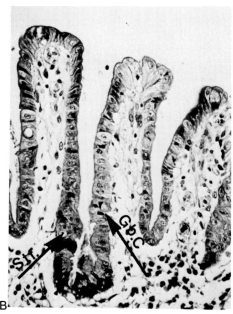

Figure 5-9. Section from resected gastric stump with carcinoma illustrates dysplasia with marked cellular atypia in intestinal metaplasia. Nuclear pleomorphism with occasional hyperchromatic, rod-shaped nuclei, nuclear stratification (Stf.), and reversed polarity of goblet cells (Gb.C) (*arrows*) are seen. Also, note the distinct brush border. H&E stain. × 80 (**A**); × 230 (**B**).

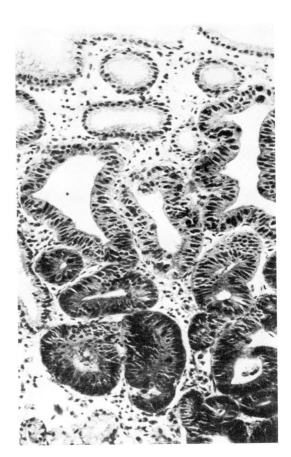

Figure 5-10. Gastroscopic biopsy from "polyp" shows all criteria for dysplasia of the intestinal type. In most areas there is still some stroma between the tubular structures. There is no definite evidence of invasion; therefore, the diagnosis was severe dysplasia of the intestinal type. When the polyp was removed, no invasive area was found. H&E stain. ×210.

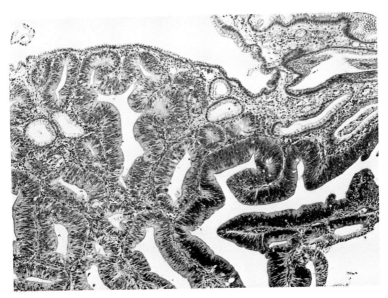

Figure 5-11. Gastroscopic biopsy from "tumor" shows very severe dysplasia of the intestinal type. Because of the marked tubular pattern of growth, the invasion is difficult to judge, but the marked back-to-back pattern favors invasive carcinoma. A repeat biopsy revealed invasive growth. H&E stain. ×80.

Table 5-1. Number of Biopsies Revealing Varying Types of Chronic
Gastritis and Dysplasia in Gastroscopic Biopsies (1977–79)

Histological Diagnosis	No. of Biopsies[a]	% of Biopsies
Chronic superficial gastritis	1,163	29.7
Chronic gastritis with varying degrees of atrophy	801	20.4
Chronic gastritis with varying degrees of atrophy and intestinal metaplasia (unqualified)	1,573	40.0
Gastritis with mild dysplasia	207	5.3
Gastritis with moderate dysplasia	109	2.8
Gastritis with severe dysplasia	68	1.8
Total number of biopsy examinations	3,921	100.0

[a]Certain patients had more than one series of biopsies. The number of patients is slightly less, therefore, than the total number of examinations. For instance, sixty-eight biopsies with severe dysplasia were taken from 40 patients.

chronic gastritis of varying degrees associated with intestinal metaplasia (unqualified) (Table 5-1).

3. It is commonly observed by pathologists working in this field that dysplasia, particularly when severe, is associated with a synchronous invasive carcinoma (19).

THE SIZE OF THE PROBLEM

The prevalence of dysplasia as defined and exemplified above is difficult to ascertain at present. This may be due partly to the short time that has passed since the publication by the WHO group of the criteria and grading of gastric dysplasia (13), and partly to the fact that pathologists tend to be rather individualistic and to stick to their "own classification." In the Department of Pathology at Ullevål Hospital, we have used the criteria largely agreed upon by the WHO group since late 1976.

During the 3-year period 1977–79 (Table 5-1), dysplasia was found in approximately 10 percent of the gastric biopsy material from patients with varying degrees of chronic gastritis and atrophy. Severe dysplasia accounted for 1.8 percent, amounting to 40 patients—a manageable group.

PRESENT SCHEME FOR FOLLOW-UP

The routine of the follow-up has changed as we have gained experience. At present we aim for the following scheme: Cases with severe dysplasia and no definite endoscopic lesion other than gastritis un-

Table 5-2. Age and Sex of Patients with Severe Dysplasia
Followed to Final Histological Diagnosis

Sex	Age (years)					Total
	30	50–59	60–69	70–79	80 +	
Male	1	3	9	10	1	24
Female	—	3	3	9	1	16
Total	1	6	12	19	2	40

dergo repeat gastroscopy with multiple biopsies (10 to 15) within 3
months. If no invasive lesion is found and there is no clinical reason
for earlier examination, repeat gastroscopy is performed with multiple biopsies every 12 months. In cases with polyps, polypectomies, or
endoscopic suspicion of malignancy, a repeat biopsy is performed as
soon as possible. In ulcer cases biopsy is repeated within 3 months
and then every 6 to 12 months.

In cases with mild and moderate dysplasia and no definite endoscopic lesion other than gastritis, biopsies are repeated within 3
months. If no more advanced lesion is found, repeat examination is
performed after 5 years.

PRELIMINARY RESULTS OF FOLLOW-UP

We felt that patients with severe dysplasia in time probably were
closer to developing cancer than patients with lesser degrees of dysplasia. Forty patients have been followed over a period of up to 5
years to a final histological diagnosis based on surgically or endoscopically removed material or at autopsy. The age and sex of the patients
in this group are presented in Table 5-2. The macroscopic lesions (en-

Table 5-3. Final Histological Diagnosis of 40 Patients with Bioptic
Diagnosis of Severe Dysplasia on First Examination

Macroscopic Lesion at Site of Biopsy	No.	No. of Carcinomas[a]	Time before Cancer Diagnosis (months)						No. of Severe Dysplasias
			3	12	24	36	48	60	
Gastritis	16	10	3	3	3	—	—	1	6
Polyp(s)[b]	10	1	—	—	1	—	—	—	9
Malignant tumor	9	9	9	—	—	—	—	—	—
Ulcer	5	2	1	—	1	—	—	—	3

[a]The 9 endoscopically recognized tumors were all advanced carcinomas; the remaining 13 were intramucosal only.

[b]The polyps were all adenomas of the tubular intestinal type.

doscopic evaluation) from which the biopsies were taken and the results of the follow-up are presented in Table 5-3.

In cases with mild and moderate dysplasia we have followed mainly patients with gastric stumps after Billroth II (B-II) resection for benign conditions, since in our country these patients form a definite high-risk group 20 to 25 years after resection (20, 21). Of approximately 60 patients followed since 1976, 2 have developed carcinoma after 5 and 6 years (Figure 5-5). Whether patients with mild and moderate dysplasia who do not belong to this group have the same risk is at present being investigated.

COMMENTS

Dysplasia as defined and described above, although not uncommon, occurs sufficiently rarely as to mark a group of patients that are more manageable for future follow-up with gastroscopy and biopsies than are patients with chronic gastritis with intestinal metaplasia. Among the patients with dysplasia, severe dysplasia is sufficiently rare to enable a very close scrutiny.

If the follow-up results of this small series of cases with severe dysplasia are representative, it can safely be concluded that this lesion is a significant precancerous or cancer-associated lesion.

The series, however, gives little in the way of information about the natural history of severe dysplasia, as it is fair to assume that at least 13 of the 22 cases that were eventually diagnosed as having carcinoma in reality represented cases of cancer-associated dysplasia.

Severe dysplasia is fairly easily recognized by the histopathologist; and if the criteria as defined above are adhered to, we should, within a comparatively short time, gather a sufficient number of cases from which to draw useful conclusions with regard to the natural history of this lesion. It is felt to be important, however, that our future study of dysplasia be linked to the endoscopic lesion with which it occurs, particularly as this also has obvious clinical implications.

Mild and moderate dysplasia offers a greater challenge, not only because the number of patients is greater, but also because of the time factor. Furthermore, the changes may be difficult to separate histologically from reactive, inflammatory changes, particularly in dysplasia of gastric epithelial origin where cellular atypia is usually less marked than in dysplasia of the intestinal type. The problem of overdiagnosis is therefore a real one.

Whereas dysplasia associated with polyps, ulcers, and "tumors" may give clinicians valuable information on which to base their patients' management, the real challenge appears to be the patient in whom dysplasia is found associated with gastritis only and in whom the endoscopist consequently has no definite focal target. This condition can be satisfactorily studied only if multiple biopsies are taken from the areas where gastritis-associated dysplasia most commonly occurs. In our experience this is in the antrum in patients with intact stomachs and on the posterior gastric wall close to the efferent loop in patients with gastric stumps after previous B-II resection.

An aphoristic hypothesis will be useful for future work: Chronic atrophic gastritis with intestinal metaplasia should be regarded as a small step on the path toward development of gastric cancer, a condition that will evolve in only a few of these patients. Dysplasia should be regarded as a big step. How big, only the future can tell.

SUMMARY

Epithelial dysplasia of the gastric mucosa is considered a precancerous lesion that should be followed by repeat examination. Compared with chronic atrophic gastritis with intestinal metaplasia, which in our department is found in 40 percent of biopsies of chronic gastritis, dysplasia is found in only 10 percent and severe dysplasia in 1.8 percent. Dysplasia therefore marks a group of patients that can be followed by repeated gastroscopies with biopsies in order to detect carcinoma at an early stage.

Forty patients with severe dysplasia were followed for up to 5 years. Twenty-four of these had a focal lesion endoscopically (10 with polyps, 9 with "tumor," and 5 with ulcer), whereas 16 had gastritis only. Twenty-two patients developed cancer or had cancer-associated dysplasia. Ten of these belonged to the group with gastritis only. All these cancers were limited to the mucosa.

Among 60 patients with lesser degrees of dysplasia, 2 developed cancer after 5 and 6 years, both diagnosed at the intramucosal stage.

The problem of follow-up is greatest in the group of patients in which the dysplasia is associated with gastritis only. We now recommend repeat biopsy within 3 months for all patients with severe and moderate dysplasia in order to detect possible cancer association. If no carcinoma is found, cases with severe dysplasia are usually followed by annual gastroscopy with multiple biopsies. Cases with lesser degrees of dysplasia can probably be left for 5 years, provided clinical features do not suggest earlier reexamination.

REFERENCES

1. Murakami, T. On the point of the development of stomach cancer. Proceeding of 19th Gen. Meeting Japan. Cancer Ass., 1960. pp. 305–312.
2. Morson, B. C. Precancerous lesions of the upper gastrointestinal tract. *JAMA* 179 (1962):311–315.
3. Ming, S.-C., Goldman, H., and Freiman, D. G. Intestinal metaplasia and histogenesis of carcinoma in human stomach. *Cancer* 20 (1967):1418–1429.
4. Correa, P., Cuello, C., and Duque, E. Carcinoma and intestinal metaplasia of the stomach in Colombian migrant. *J. Natl. Cancer Inst.* 44 (1970):297–306.
5. Nagayo, T. Histological diagnosis of biopsied gastric mucosa with special reference to that of borderline lesions. *Gann Monogr. Cancer Res.* 11 (1972): 245–256.
6. Schade, R. O. K. The borderline between benign and malignant lesions in the stomach. In *Early Gastric Cancer. Current Status of Diagnosis*, edited by Grundmann, E., Grunze, H., and Witte, S., pp. 45–53. Berlin: Springer-Verlag, 1974.
7. Eder, M. Problems of formal genesis of carcinoma of the stomach. In *Early Gastric Cancer. Current Status of Diagnosis*, edited by Grundmann, E., Grunze, H., and Witte, S., pp. 27–33. Berlin: Springer-Verlag, 1974.
8. Oehlert, W., Keller, P., Henke, M., and Strach, M. Die Dysplasien der Magenschleimhaut. *Dtsch. Med. Wochenschr.* 100 (1975):150–159.
9. Grundmann, E. Histological types and possible initial stages in early gastric carcinoma. *Beitr. Pathol.* 154 (1975):256–280.
10. Ming, S.-C. Gastric carcinoma. A pathobiological classification. *Cancer* 39 (1977):2475–2485.
11. Nagayo, T. Early histogenesis of human gastric carcinoma. In *Gastric Cancer. Etiology and Pathogenesis*, edited by Pfeiffer, C. J., pp. 128–138. New York: G. Witztrock, 1979.
12. Grundmann, E., and Schlake, W. Histological classification of gastric cancer from initial to advanced stages. *Pathol. Res. Pract.* 173 (1982):260–274.
13. Morson, B. C., Sobin, L. H., Grundmann, E., Johansen, A., Nagayo, T., and Serck-Hanssen, A. Precancerous conditions and epithelial dysplasia in the stomach. *J. Clin. Pathol.* 33 (1980):711–721.
14. World Health Organization. Report of a WHO meeting on the Histological Definition of Precancerous Lesions. Geneva: WHO, 1972.
15. Järvi, O., and Laurén, P. On the role of heterotopias of the intestinal epithelium in the pathogenesis of gastric cancer. *Acta Pathol. Microbiol. Scand.* 29 (1951):26–44.
16. Morson, B. C. Carcinoma arising from areas of intestinal metaplasia in the gastric mucosa. *Br. J. Cancer* 9 (1955):377–385.
17. Siurala, M., Varis, K., and Wilasalo, M. Studies of patients with atrophic gastritis: A 10–15 year follow-up. *Scand. J. Gastroenterol.* 1 (1966):40–48.
18. Siurala, M., Lehtola, J., and Thamäki, T. Atrophic gastritis and its sequelae. Results of 19–23 years of follow-up examinations. *Scand. J. Gastroenterol.* 9 (1974):441–446.
19. Serck-Hanssen, A. Histopathology. In *Early Gastric Cancer. Proceedings of the Second BSG. SK&F International Workshop*, edited by Cotton, P. B., pp. 45–48. London: Smith Kline & French Lab. Ltd., 1982.

20. Stalsberg, H., and Taksdal, S. Stomach cancer following gastric surgery for be-
    nign conditions. *Lancet* 2 (1971):1175–1177.
21. Schrumpf, E., Serck-Hanssen, A., Stadaas, J., Aune, S., Myren, J., and Osnes, M.
    Mucosal changes in the gastric stump 20–25 years after partial gastrectomy. *Lan-
    cet* 2 (1977):467–469.

6 PRENEOPLASTIC LESIONS OF THE STOMACH

W. Oehlert

The definition and identification of precancerous lesions in the stomach are based primarily on the specific histological changes in the vicinity of carcinomas. In pioneering studies by Büchner (1) and von Konjetzny (2), it was suggested that the changes of the mucosa preceded the onset of tumor growth. These observations allow a broad interpretation as a precancerous lesion of histological changes adjacent to a carcinoma. However, by strictly adhering to the definition of this specific lesion, only those histological changes that are irreversible and that predict the development of a carcinoma within the patient's normal life span should be considered precancerous.

As long as the description and evaluation of histological changes were limited to resected specimens alone, considerations regarding the reversibility of these specific changes were of mere theoretical interest. The situation is entirely different when we consider the diagnostic significance of the specific changes in the biopsy material, calling for appropriate measures to be taken by the clinician. This is one of the reasons for introducing the definitions of precancerous condition and precancerous change into international usage, as suggested by Nagayo (3). Table 6-1 shows that the histological changes occurring frequently in biopsy material can be attributed to either precancerous

Table 6-1.   Precancerous Lesions of the Stomach

Precancerous Lesions	Pathologic Diagnosis	Prognosis	Therapy
Precancerous condition	Atrophic gastritis; intestinal metaplasia; enterocolic metaplasia; hyperplasiogenic polyp	Development of a carcinoma possible, but not safely predictable; underlying lesion for precancerous changes	No invasive therapy
Precancerous change	Dysplasia III; adenomatous polyp with atypias	Development of a carcinoma probable—prospective period unknown	Removal of all polypoid lesions absolutely mandatory

conditions or precancerous changes. As a consequence, the clinician is required to remove every polypoid lesion from the stomach, lest subsequent histological investigations reveal clearly tumorous changes. Polypoid lesions should be distinguished from genuine gastric polyps and other benign changes, such as mucosal cysts, hyperplastic polyps, and polypoid foveolar hyperplasias. Since polypoid changes of the gastric mucosa are also produced by some severe dysplasias and special forms of early gastric carcinoma, it is advisable to remove all polypoid lesions surgically (Table 6-2). Other lesions that spread laterally or are multiple cannot be removed in this simple way. These lesions still present considerable problems to both the pathologist and the clinician as regards establishing the diagnosis, determining the prognosis, and instituting a suitable therapy.

Based on our own findings, obtained by means of proliferation kinetics and cytophotometric and immunohistochemical investigations, we have proposed the designation "dysplasia" for specific disturbances in the differentiation of the superficial epithelium, showing a possible precancerous tendency (4). We have further suggested a grading system to subdivide dysplasia into three different forms, which are practically identical to the forms of dysplasia defined by Grundmann (5) and Ming (6). Table 6-3 shows the histological features and proliferation kinetics characterizing the different degrees of severity of dysplasia. Figures 6-1 and 6-2 give examples of the histological picture of dysplasia II and III.

Our definition of dysplasia III, which Ming (6) described as dysplasia IV and Grundmann (5) as severe dysplasia, almost completely conforms to the definitions of borderline lesion, intraepithelial carcinoma, and superficial spreading carcinoma (7–10).

Table 6-2. Polypoid Nonneoplastic and Neoplastic Changes
of Gastric Mucosa

Change	Diagnosis	Therapy	Additional Measures
Epithelial nonneoplastic			
Cysts of gastric glands	Biopsy	—	—
Heterotopic pancreatic tissue	Biopsy	—	—
Patchy foveolar hyperplasia	Biopsy	—	—
Patchy polypoid foveolar hyperplasia	Biopsy	—	—
Hyperplastic (hyperplasiogenous) polyp	Biopsy	Endoscopic polypectomy	—
Mesenchymal nonneoplastic			
Fibroid polyp	Biopsy	—	—
Pseudolymphoma	Biopsy	—	Endoscopic polypectomy for final diagnosis
Epithelial neoplastic			
Adenomatous polyp (villoglandular adenoma)	Biopsy	Endoscopic excision	—
Villous polyp or adenoma	Biopsy	Endoscopic excision	Follow-ups
Adenomatous dysplasia III	Biopsy	Endoscopic excision	Follow-ups
Early cancer (elevated type)	Biopsy (preliminary diagnosis)	Endoscopic excision (if possible)	Follow-ups or gastrectomy
Carcinoids	Biopsy	Endoscopic excision	Follow-ups
Mesenchymal neoplastic			
Leiomyoma	Biopsy	Surgical removal	—
Myoblastoma	Biopsy	Surgical removal	—
Leiomyosarcoma	Biopsy	Operation + irradiation	Follow-ups
Neurinoma	Biopsy	Operation	Follow-ups
Malignant lymphoma	Biopsy (preliminary diagnosis)	—	Endoscopic excision for final diagnosis or classification
Lipoma	Biopsy	—	—

Table 6-3. Cell Proliferation Kinetics, Nuclear Diameter, and DNA Content
in the Normal and Abnormal Epithelia of the Stomach

	Condition of the Epithelium				
	Normal	Inflammation	Atrophic Gastritis	Dysplasia III	Early Cancer
Mean lifetime (days)	8–20	2.7–4.5	1.25	1.0	1.0
Nuclear diameter (μm)	5.8–7.9	—	7.9–10.5	10.0–15.0	8.0–15.0
DNA content (%)					
$2n$	90	—	50–75	—	20–50
$3–4n$	10	—	25–50	—	50–80

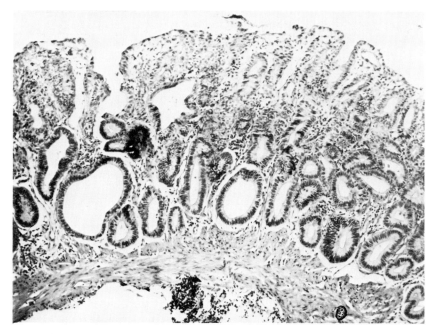

Figure 6-1. Dysplasia II of the surface epithelium in a case of chronic atrophic gastritis. The gastric foveolae are transformed into glandular formations lined by epithelial cells, which are no longer mucigenous, and contain clearly pleomorphic nuclei. The depletion of mucus formation has led to small, superficial erosions and inflammatory infiltration of the stroma. H&E stain. × 10.

As illustrated in Table 6-4, our test results, gained from a large patient group over a period of 4 years, have revealed that the histological changes defined as dysplasia are basically reversible, that they sometimes persist with the same degree of severity, but that in only rare cases do they transform into a carcinoma. Our findings were confirmed by Potet and Camilleri (11) who conducted similar experiments over a 4-year period. The question arises as to whether the use of structural, histochemical, or immunohistochemical methods permits conclusions to be drawn concerning the tendency of severe dysplasia to progress to malignancy. Neither proliferation kinetics, nor cytophotometric measurements, nor histochemical investigations of the mucus have been helpful in indicating the further development of this lesion.

Wurster and Rapp (12) reported a positive correlation between the cellular atypia, the production of carcinoembryonic antigen (CEA), and the degree of severity of the dysplasia. We had hoped that the presence of CEA would help in obtaining further differentiation of severe dysplasia. CEA in the cells of various forms of dysplasia that we

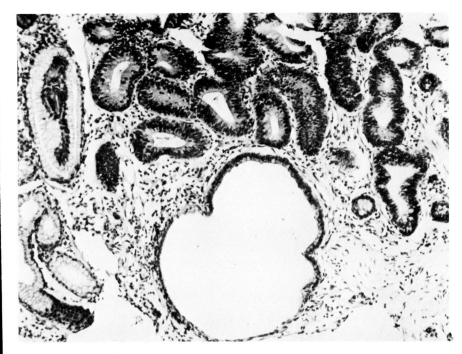

Figure 6-2. Dysplasia III of the surface epithelium in chronic atrophic gastritis accompanied by enterocolic metaplasia of the surrounding epithelium. The gastric foveolae are transformed into glandular formations, produce hardly any mucus, and show densely packed pleomorphic nuclei. Enterocolic metaplasia can be recognized at the left margin, and a mucous cyst is seen in the center. H&E stain. × 10.

Table 6-4. Follow-Up of Dysplasias II and III in Biopsy Specimens

Dysplasia at Initial Diagnosis	No. of Patients	Reexamination after	Status		
			Improved	Unchanged	Deteriorated
II	672 (100%)	2–12 months	437 (65.03%)	211 (31.40%)	24 (3.50%)
III	498 (100%)		371 (74.50%)	127 (25.50%)	—·
II	268 (100%)	1–2 years	107 (39.93%)	150 (55.97%)	11 (4.10%)
III	121 (100%)		61 (50.40%)	60 (49.60%)	—
II	96 (100%)	2–3 years	32 (33.40%)	44 (45.80%)	20 (20.80%)
III	152 (100%)		35 (23.00%)	117 (77.00%)	—
II	12 (100%)	>3 years	—	12 (100.0%)	—
III	46 (100%)		7 (15.30%)	35 (76.00%)	4 (8.70%) early cancer

have investigated in our department did not, unfortunately, allow reliable conclusions to be drawn as to the reversibility or irreversibility of the process of dysplasia.

We must therefore be aware that the use of even the most recent cytophotometric and histochemical methods will not permit the prediction of the growth tendency of severe dysplasia. As a result, the identification of dysplasia III will not entail any therapeutic consequences, but will require an immediate, thorough check-up, which may reveal a carcinoma that escaped notice at the time of the first biopsy. Moreover, we would like to advise clinicians to continue to examine the patients at intervals of 3 to 6 months.

This type of dysplasia III of the superficial epithelium of the gastric mucosa may be considered a preliminary stage of the intestinal type of gastric carcinoma, but no prediction can be made regarding the period during which the lesion is expected to develop into a carcinoma.

In most cases of signet-ring cell or the diffuse type of gastric carcinomas, the superficial epithelium does not show any dysplastic changes (13). Signet-ring cell carcinomas, occurring at an ever-increasing rate in the region of the fundus of both male and female young adults, frequently develop without being accompanied either by atrophic gastritis or by intestinal or enterocolic metaplasia. On the other hand, the conspicuous changes observed regularly in the mucus-forming epithelial cells of the superficial part of the tumor warrant their diagnostic significance, even though a fully developed carcinoma has not yet been identified.

In the initial stage, some cells of the superficial epithelium, usually lying near the neck of a gland, are arranged in a different manner and show a rounded appearance (Figure 6-3). In the second phase of development, the gastric foveolae form protrusions as a result of the accumulation of round cells, in which the coarse, granular mucus replaces the fine, granular one. In these foci a different type of mucus can be observed, which shows a steadily decreasing positive reaction for periodic acid-Schiff stain. In contrast, the new type of mucus stains increasingly well with alcian blue. A further reduction in the typical cell formation within the area of the superficial epithelium is accompanied by an inflammatory reaction in the vicinity of these cells. Immunohistochemical investigations, using antibodies against CEA linked to peroxidase, revealed that CEA is rarely seen in the rounded cells still lying within the epithelial walls, but is almost always found in those lying outside. These cells, showing a different appearance and stainability, are largely identical to the three types of signet-

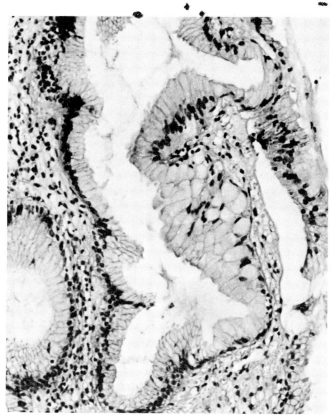

Figure 6-3.   Beginning dysplasia of mucus formation in the surface epithelium of the gastric mucosa. The regular basement membrane of the tall cylindrical epithelium is lost (**right**). Round mucigenous cells with a finely granular cytoplasm are present in the same part of the picture. The positive reaction of the round cells with alcian blue stain (AB) reflects production of acid mucopolysaccharides. The typical surface epithelial cells give a negative reaction with AB and stain positively with periodic acid-Schiff stain. H&E stain. × 360.

ring cells identified with electron microscopy by Yamashiro and coworkers (14; Figure 6-4). The changes reported in our study were defined before by Cain and Kraus (15), who used the term "carcinoma in situ of the stomach." Schlake and Grundmann (16) described similar changes as an initial stage of signet-ring cell carcinoma, and Schauer and Kunze (17) were able to confirm the changes, observed in our biopsy material, in *N*-methyl-*N'*-nitro-*N*-nitrosoguanidine-induced carcinomas of the stomach in rats.

In 1979 Watanabe and coworkers (18) induced carcinoma in the dog by administering *N*-nitroso-butylurea. They interpreted the disturbed maturation of mucus-forming cells within the gastric foveolae

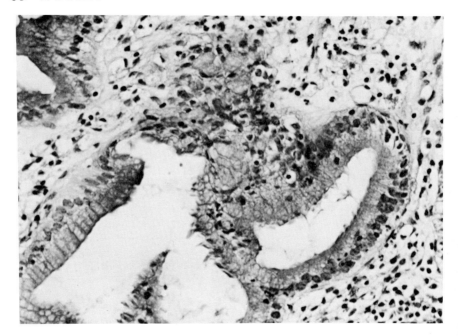

Figure 6-4.   Severe dysplasia of mucus production associated with signet-ring cell formation. In addition to the round appearance of the epithelial cells (shown in Figure 3), some isolated round cells with a coarsely vacuolar cytoplasm and marginal nuclei lie outside the basement membrane and are surrounded by inflammatory cells. H&E stain. × 400.

as an early change indicating carcinogenesis. During this process, rounded, mucus-forming cells are transferred into the lamina propria.

On the basis of the current data, it can be assumed that a disturbed formation of mucus in the area of gastric foveolae is to be considered an early change in carcinogenesis that may develop further either into a signet-ring cell or the diffuse type of gastric carcinoma. So far, no extensive control tests are available that could give information concerning the various stages of development toward the so-called carcinoma in situ and whether these stages are to be considered reversible or irreversible. Nothing is known about the period of time during which these mucosal changes eventually transform into early or fully developed carcinoma. As in the case of dysplasia III, the pathologist must ask the clinician to perform necessary medical examinations. We feel that owing to the currently existing uncertainty regarding a possible progression of these changes, the term "carcinoma in situ" should be avoided, because this definition entails surgical intervention. We therefore prefer to describe this condition as a disturbed mucus formation similar to the description of the dysplasias of

Table 6-5. Dysplasias of Gastric Mucosa and Their Clinical Significance

Diagnosis	Local Changes and Accompanying Symptoms	Suggestions for Follow-up to the Clinician
Dysplasia I Regenerating epithe- lium without atypia	Surface gastritis Chronic gastritis Atrophy Erosion Edge of gastric ulcer Billroth II anastomosis (<10 years)	All cases: Not required
Dysplasia II Mitotically active epi- thelium with atypia	Surface gastritis Chronic gastritis Atrophy	Not required
	Ulcer scar Erosion Edge of gastric ulcer	Control of healing every 2 years
	Billroth II anastomosis (>10 years)	Once a year
Dysplasia III Mitotically active epi- thelium with atypia and transformation	Surface gastritis Chronic gastritis Atrophy Ulcer scar Erosion Edge of gastric ulcer Billroth II anastomosis	All cases: *Immediately* fol- lowed by regular check-ups every 6 months

various degrees. We hope that thorough and regular medical check-ups will make further information available.

Based on the current knowledge of precancerous changes of the gastric mucosa, our feeling is that after recognizing the different forms of dysplasia, suggestions for further procedures shown in Table 6-5 should be made available to the clinician.

REFERENCES

1. Büchner, F. Die Pathologie der peptischen Varanderungen und ihre Beziehung zum Magenkarzinom. *Veroeff. Kriegspathol. Konstitutionspathol.* 18 (1927): 1–125.
2. von Konjetzny, G. E. *Der Magenkrebs.* Stuttgart: Enke Verlag, 1938.
3. Nagayo, T. Precursors of human gastric cancer: Their frequencies and histological characteristics. In *Pathophysiology of Carcinogenesis in Digestive Organs,* edited by Farber, E., pp. 151–161. Tokyo: University of Tokyo Press, 1977.

4. Oehlert, W., Keller, P., Henke, M., and Strauch, M. Die Dysplasien der Magenschleimhaut. Das Problem inihrer klinischen Bedeutung. *Dtsch. Med. Wochenschr.* 100 (1975):1950.

5. Grundmann, E. Histologic types and possible initial stages in early gastric carcinoma. *Beitr. Pathol.* 154 (1975):256–280.

6. Ming, S.-C. Dysplasia of gastric epithelium. *Front. Gastrointest. Res.* 4 (1979):164–172.

7. Elster, K., and Kudlich, W. Die diagnostische Effektivität der Gastrobiopsie. *Endoscopy* 4 (1972):162.

8. Nagayo, T. Microscopical cancer of the stomach. A study on histogenesis of gastric carcinoma. *Int. J. Cancer* 16 (1975):52–60.

9. Schade, R.O.K. The borderline between benign and malignant lesions in the stomach. In *Early Gastric Cancer. Current Status of Diagnosis*, edited by Grundmann, E., Grunze, H., and Witte, S., p. 45. Berlin: Springer-Verlag, 1974.

10. Crespi, M., Bigotti, A., and di Matteo, S. Early gastric cancer. In *Early Gastric Cancer. Current Status of Diagnosis*, edited by Grundmann, E., Grunze, H., and Witte, S., p. 60. Berlin: Springer-Verlag, 1974.

11. Potet, F., and Camilleri, J. P. Population à haut risque et dysplasia précancereuses de l'estomac: Définition et attitude pratique. *Gastroenterol. Clin. Biol.* 6 (1982):454–461.

12. Wurster, K., and Rapp, W. Histological and immunohistological studies on gastric mucosa. I. The presence of CEA in dysplastic surface epithelium. *Pathol. Res. Pract.* 164 (1979):270–281.

13. Cuello, C., and Correa, P. Dysplastic changes in intestinal metaplasia of the gastric mucosa. In *Gastric Cancer*, edited by Herfarth, Ch., and Schlag, P., pp. 83–90. Berlin: Springer-Verlag, 1979.

14. Yamashiro, K., Suzuki, H., and Nagayo, T. Electron microscopic study of signet ring cells in diffuse carcinoma of the human stomach. *Virchows Arch. (Pathol. Anat.)* 374 (1977):275–284.

15. Cain, H., and Kraus, B. Frühkarzinom des Magens. *Dtsch. Med. Wochenschr.* 98 (1973):1591–1596.

16. Schlake, W., and Grundmann, E. Multifocal early gastric cancer of mixed type. *Pathol. Res. Pract.* 164 (1979):331–341.

17. Schauer, A., and Kunze, E. Relation of adenomatous hyperplasia of the gastric mucosa to carcinogenesis. *Pathol. Res. Pract.* 164 (1979):238–248.

18. Watanabe, H., Hirose, F., Kakizawa, S., Terada, Y., Fujii, I., and Ohkita, T. A mode of incipient growth in chemically induced signet ring cell carcinoma of the canine stomach. *Pathol. Res. Pract.* 164 (1979):216–223.

7 GASTRIC MUCOSAL DYSPLASIA: PRELIMINARY RESULTS OF A PROSPECTIVE STUDY OF PATIENTS FOLLOWED FOR PERIODS OF UP TO SIX YEARS

J. P. Camilleri, F. Potet, C. Amat, and G. Molas

The natural history of epithelial dysplasia in the stomach remains largely unknown, and the degree of risk associated with this condition is not yet established. Most investigations based on biopsy or operation material have been retrospective (1–8). A close follow-up of such patients including endoscopic biopsies must be initiated in order to provide new insights in this field (9–11).

In view of this, in 1976 we started a systematic prospective study of epithelial dysplasia in the stomach, and we are now presenting the preliminary results of a follow-up period of up to 6 years.

PATIENTS AND METHODS

Our study was based on biopsy material from the Departments of Pathology of Broussais and Beaujon Hospitals in Paris.

The initial series consisted of 12,394 gastric biopsies performed in patients during the years 1976–82. All the specimens were fixed in Bouin's fluid and embedded in paraffin. Five-micron sections at two or three levels were cut and stained with hematoxylin-eosin-safran (HES).

All the histological material was carefully examined with regard to the presence or absence of epithelial dysplasia. Gastric polyps were not included in this study. For patients in whom dysplastic epithelial changes were found, we asked the clinician for reendoscopy within 6 months, irrespective of the concomitant disease of the gastric mucosa. In patients with ulcer, six or more specimens were taken at the edge of each lesion. In patients with prior gastric resection, specimens were taken from around the stoma as well as from elsewhere in the stomach, usually the lesser curve. In patients with diffuse gastritis, ten or more specimens were taken from the suspicious area and further specimens from any lesion seen. The slides were reviewed by at least two of us to arrive at a final grading of the lesion. When a dysplasia was demonstrated in such biopsy material, a follow-up of the patient at 1-year intervals was required. For patients who were operated on, the resection specimens were cut into thin slices and several sections from any macroscopic changes were examined.

GRADING OF EPITHELIAL DYSPLASIA

The idea of follow-up study needs a precise definition of the term "dysplasia" in biopsy material.

The first task for the pathologist must be to separate the dysplastic from the regenerative and/or hyperplastic changes. An increased regenerative activity of the surface epithelium, whatever the cause, is manifested by an enlargement of nuclear diameter with a shift in the nuclear-cytoplasmic ratio, a reduced mucus production in the whole gastric pit, and a raised mitotic number. This structural transformation of the gastric pits is capable of rapid regression, and must be distinguished from dysplasia, which means disorder of growth with an increased malignant potential.

According to the World Health Organization (WHO) recommendations, epithelial dysplasia refers to the following histological and

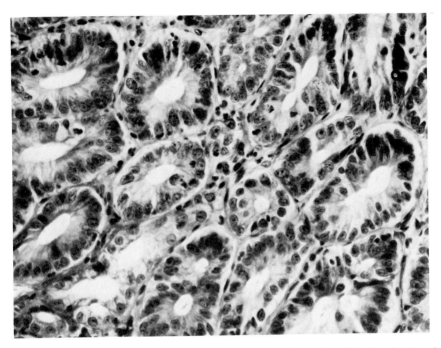

Figure 7-1.   Moderate dysplasia. The tubules are packed together. The dysplastic epithelium shows loss of mucus secretion, enlargement of nuclei, and shift in the nuclear-cytoplasmic ratio. HES stain. × 300.

cytological criteria: abnormal cytology, abnormal differentiation, and abnormal architecture. So, both cytological and architectural changes are needed for the diagnosis of epithelial dysplasia. Sometimes cellular atypias can be seen in regenerative-hyperplastic changes, whereas intestinal metaplasia of the incomplete type may show some architectural disarray without marked cytological atypia.

In the present work, grading of dysplasia was limited to moderate and severe grades. Moderate dysplasia was composed of crowded, dark, basophilic cells, with substantial loss of mucus secretion; tubules usually were packed together in rather close contact (Figure 7-1). Sometimes the cells were not dark, even pale, when mucus secretion persisted, and in such cases the diagnosis of dysplasia was difficult and based mainly on nuclear abnormalities. Inverted goblet cells could be found. In severe dysplasia the abnormal architecture was more marked, with abnormal budding or branching, back-to-back fusion, and papillary infolding; cellular atypia displayed nuclear hyperchromatism and pleomorphism; and many nuclei shifted to-

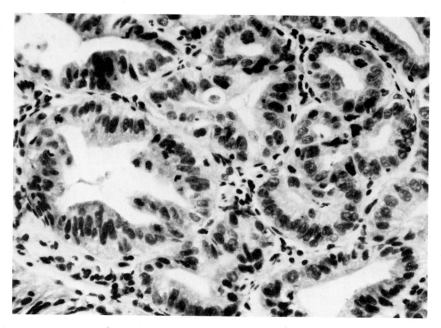

Figure 7-2.   Severe dysplasia. Irregular, branched epithelial structures show marked nuclear pleomorphism. HES stain. ×300.

ward the lumen and piled on top. The degree of pseudostratification was variable (Figures 7-2 and 7-3).

In some cases development of epithelial buds led to frank adenomatous transformation, comprising closely packed tubular proliferation of columnar cells, with pseudostratified, rod-shaped, hyperchromatic nuclei (Figure 7-3).

Finally, severe epithelial dysplasia must be distinguished from intramucosal carcinoma, the latter term being used only when lamina propria invasion can be documented. So, examination of multiple sections through the tissue is essential, and it is impossible to be sure that small groups of tumor cells have not crossed the epithelial basement membrane. The terms "carcinoma in situ" and "preinvasive cancer" have been avoided in this work.

Table 7-1.   Gastric Lesions Associated with Dysplasia in 327 Patients

Gastric Lesions	No.	%
Ulcers	115	35.16
Diffuse gastritis	169	51.68
Gastric stumps	43	13.14

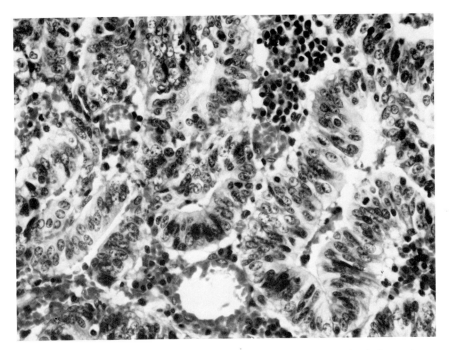

Figure 7-3.   Severe dysplasia. Adenomatous tubules with back-to-back formation are present. The dysplastic epithelium shows pseudostratification with multiple rows of nuclei that shift toward the lumen and marked nuclear hyperchromatism and pleomorphism. HES stain. × 300.

RESULTS OF THE FIRST BIOPSY

In a total of 12,394 gastric biopsies performed in the two departments, gastric mucosal dysplasia was found in 464 biopsies (3.75 percent) in 327 patients: 34 (0.27 percent) with severe dysplasia and 430 (3.47 percent) with moderate dysplasia. The average age of the patients was 55 years (range 28 to 83 years). The ratio of females to males was 1:3.6.

As shown in Table 7-1, 35.16 percent of the dysplasias were found at the edge of ulcers, 51.68 percent in diffuse gastritis, and 13.14 percent in gastric stumps after partial resection. Our study has not covered gastric polyps.

Of the 327 patients, the initial grading was severe dysplasia in 24 and moderate dysplasia in 303. When patients underwent reendoscopy within 6 months, changes for the worse were taken into account to arrive at the grading of the lesion.

Table 7-2. Follow-Up of Severe Dysplasia (24 Patients)

Status	No. of Patients
Operated (8 patients)	
Early carcinoma	3
Advanced carcinoma	3
Severe dysplasia	2
Nonoperated (16 patients)	
No follow-up	6
Followed	10
<6 months	5
1–3 years	5
Unchanged	3
Regressed	2

RESULTS OF FOLLOW-UP STUDIES

In 24 patients with severe dysplasia (Table 7-2), 8 were operated on within 2 years. Early gastric carcinoma was diagnosed in three and advanced carcinoma in three. In two no invasive carcinoma was found, and histological examination of multiple sections from the suspicious areas showed a wide range of appearances, including varying degrees of chronic atrophic gastritis, intestinal metaplasia, and foci of moderate to severe dysplasia. Among the nonoperated patients, six did not reply and five underwent their first endoscopy within the last 6 months of the study. Five patients were followed over periods of up to 3 years. Our control examinations showed that histological grading of epithelial changes remained unchanged in three cases, but regressed from severe to moderate dysplasia or regenerative-hyperplastic changes in two. In one patient who had been followed over 3 years, six gastric biopsies continued to show severe dysplastic changes.

All patients with moderate dysplasia were requested for a systematic reexamination at 1-year intervals. One hundred fifty-seven patients (51 percent) declined to be reexamined or did not reply; 14 were operated on for ulcer disease, and discontinuous moderate dysplastic changes were found in the surgically resected specimens. In the remaining 132 patients, 28 had their first endoscopy within the last 6 months of the study. One hundred one patients were surveyed for a follow-up period of 1 to 6 years. In 47 patients no dysplasia was found at the time of reexamination after a follow-up period ranging from 1 to 5 years. In 54 patients dysplastic changes were found in one or more repeated biopsies. For these patients details of the histologi-

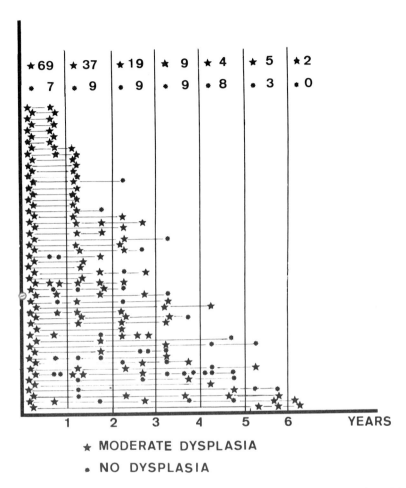

★ MODERATE DYSPLASIA

• NO DYSPLASIA

Figure 7-4.   Details of survey in 54 patients with moderate dysplasia in the initial as well as in one or more follow-up biopsies (190 total). Biopsies of the same patients are indicated by horizontal lines.

cal findings are shown in Figure 7-4. In many cases histological appearances varied from one examination to another. In a total of 190 biopsies, no dysplasia was found in 45 (23 percent). With regard to the period of the survey, the number of biopsies without dysplasia is given in Figure 7-4. According to our findings, the proportion of negative biopsies appeared to increase with the time of the survey; however, the absence of dysplastic appearances in follow-up biopsies did not necessarily mean that the histological changes had regressed, but perhaps that the lesions suspected of dysplasia had escaped from the biopsy. Only one asymptomatic patient had a broad-based soft polyp 4 years after the first endoscopy; multiple biopsies showed moderate dysplasia associated with adenomatous changes. No progression from moderate to severe dysplasia was found in this series.

DISCUSSION

The grading of dysplasia has been widely discussed in the past 10 years (3, 5, 7, 9, 10). According to the general agreement at the WHO meeting in 1978, Morson et al. (6) divided the epithelial changes into mild, moderate, and severe dysplasia. It is clear that mild dysplasia is a common finding in the diseased stomach, notably in benign conditions. It probably represents excessive regeneration of acute or chronic cell loss, and would be better called regenerative-hyperplastic epithelial changes. The term "dysplasia" means disorder of growth and differentiation and needs both architectural and cellular atypias to be documented. As far as the gastric mucosa is concerned, it seems that dysplasia is perhaps overdiagnosed.

Recently, two types of dysplasia have been described with regard to the type of cellular differentiation; types I and II of Jass (2) would correspond to the adenomatous and hyperplastic types of Cuello et al. (1). The former is the more classic type, found mainly in tubular adenomas. Since polypoid lesions were not included in our study, this type of dysplasia was not frequently observed in this series. However, both types can arise in endoscopically flat mucosa, and may coexist in the same specimen. Whether the natural history of each type of dysplasia is different remains unknown, particularly concerning their ability to acquire enough mass to form true polyps. In our material such transformation was noted in only one patient.

Little is known of the incidence of gastric dysplasia. Several data reported in the literature are based on the study of gastric mucosa surrounding overt neoplasms, another reason that advanced dysplastic changes may be overestimated. Our material consisted of randomly collected gastric biopsies from patients seemingly without clinical or endoscopic suspicion of cancer. Under these circumstances the incidence of gastric dysplasia was in the same range as in the prospective series of Oehlert et al. (9, 10). In this study the average age of patients with gastric dysplasia was lower than that of patients with carcinoma. If the frequency of dysplasia is now related to different concomitant gastric diseases, our results were in agreement with the data available in the medical literature (6, 10).

It is generally thought that severe dysplasia is linked to an increased malignant potential. Previous investigations have shown that, in contrast to the lower grade of dysplasia, only severe dysplasia occurs more frequently in carcinoma cases than in benign cases (4, 5). According to our findings, severe dysplasia was associated with gastric carcinoma in at least one-third of the cases. It is of interest that, in our series, early carcinoma was found in three of eight resected stomachs. Therefore, since the precise grading of histological appearances is sometimes uncertain, the primary task is to search for a coexisting carcinoma. If there is no tumor, the management of individual cases remains a matter of debate. Up to now, severe dysplasia by itself has not been an indication for surgery. In the course of this study, the transition of severe dysplasia to early gastric cancer has not yet been observed. However, in 46 patients followed for more than 3 years, Oehlert et al. (10) were able to find such transition in 4 cases. The heterogeneity of the histological findings from one examination to another probably reflects the difficulty of detecting multiple and discontinuous changes in flat mucosa. Such cases deserve repeated multiple biopsies taken precisely in the suspicious areas.

All patients with moderate dysplasia need to be carefully checked at regular intervals. Such routine follow-up study is always compromised by the difficulty in surveying asymptomatic patients over a long period of time. In our study only 49 percent of patients accepted screening. Patients with a chronic ulcer scar as well as patients who have had a partial gastrectomy should be controlled more easily than patients with diffuse gastritis. In this series obvious progression of moderate to severe dysplasia could not be documented in any case, and only one patient displayed transformation to a polypoid lesion during the survey period. It is probable that dysplasia could regress in some cases, as shown by the increasing number of negative biopsies with time. Nevertheless, we must be aware of the fact that suspicious areas can escape from the biopsy. So it is necessary to keep all patients in whom dysplasia has been found under review. The results depend on the experience of the endoscopist, and close cooperation between clinician and pathologist is needed.

ACKNOWLEDGMENTS

This work was carried out on material collected at the Departments of Endoscopy of Broussais Hospital (J. P. Petite, F. Bloch) and Beaujon Hospital (J. A. Paolaggi, C. Theodore). We are indebted to our clinical colleagues for their help and their most useful advice. We thank also M. Wolfelsperger for photographic help and S. Peyret for typing the manuscript.

REFERENCES

1. Cuello, C., Correa, P., Zarama, G., Copez, J., Murray, J., and Gordillo, G. Histopathology of gastric dysplasias. *Am. J. Surg. Pathol.* 3 (1975):491–500.
2. Jass, J. R. A classification of gastric dysplasia. *Histopathology* 7 (1983):181–193.
3. Grundmann, E. Histologic types and possible initial stages in early gastric carcinoma. *Beitr. Pathol.* 154 (1975):256–280.
4. Meister, H., Holubarsch, C. H., Haferkamp, O., Schlag, P., and Herfarth, Ch. Gastritis, intestinal metaplasia and dysplasia versus benign ulcer in stomach and duodenum and gastric carcinoma. *Pathol. Res. Pract.* 164 (1979):259–269.
5. Ming, S.-C. Dysplasia of gastric epithelium. *Front. Gastrointest. Res.* 4 (1979):164–172.
6. Morson, B. C., Sobin, L. H., Grundmann, E., Johansen, A., Nagayo, T., and Serck-Hanssen, A. Precancerous condition and epithelial dysplasia in the stomach. *Clin. Pathol.* 33 (1980):711–721.
7. Nagayo, T. Histological diagnosis of biopsied gastric mucosa with special reference to that of borderline lesions. *Gann Monogr. Cancer Res.* 11 (1971):245–256.
8. Schade, R. O. K. The borderline between benign and malignant lesions in the stomach. In *Early Gastric Cancer*, edited by Grundmann, E., Gruntze, H., and Witte, S., pp. 45–53. Berlin: Springer-Verlag, 1974.
9. Oehlert, W., Keller, P., Henke, M., and Stauch, M. Die Dysplasien der Magenschleimhaut. *Dtsch. Med. Wochenschr.* 100 (1975):1950–1956.
10. Oehlert, W., Keller, P., Henke, M., and Strauch, M. Gastric mucosal dysplasia: What is its clinical significance? *Front. Gastrointest. Res.* 4 (1979):173–182.
11. Siurala, M., and Salmi, H. J. Long term follow-up of subjects with superficial gastritis and a normal gastric mucosa. *Scand. J. Gastroenterol.* 6 (1971):459–463.

8 METAPLASIA, DYSPLASIA, AND EARLY GASTRIC CANCER

K. Elster, M. Stolte, W. Carson, and H. Eidt

Whether you are reading a pathological or histological report or are studying a clinical paper that deals with stomach cancer, you will always find the terms "metaplasia," "dysplasia," and "early gastric cancer." Perhaps you have gotten angry about the fact that these concepts are often interpreted differently and not seldom are misleading. We believe that it will be helpful before discussing this subject to define the terms clearly.

DEFINITION OF TERMS

Metaplasia means a change of one sort of tissue into another sort. In relation to gastric mucosa, one speaks of intestinal metaplasia if the mucosa has structures like the small bowel, with villi and crypts and glands with goblet and Paneth cells, much like the mucosa of the small bowel. Enterocolic metaplasia (1) is a variant of intestinal metaplasia; that is, with an increase in the number of goblet cells, there is a similarity to large bowel structure (Figure 8-1). This intestinal metaplasia may

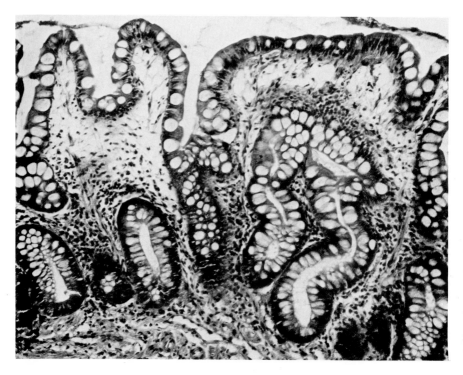

Figure 8-1.   Biopsy specimen shows intestinal metaplasia, partly of the enterocolic type. H&E stain. × 200.

be considered a normal finding in prepyloric areas, at the border of the body and antrum, and in the cardiac mucosa.

Dysplasia is defined as cellular atypia, abnormal differentiation, and disorganized mucosal architecture (Figure 8-2).

We need not define the subgroups of these terms, for in their various versions they are confusing even for the histologist (2–6).

An early gastric cancer is a carcinoma of the stomach in which invasion is limited to the mucosa and submucosa. It should be emphasized that this diagnosis may be made only in a preparation in which all layers of the stomach wall are found; this means, in most cases, after resection (Figure 8-3).

Thinking about these definitions, and letting these topics with several concepts pass before the eyes, one may be tempted to suppose that there is a sequence. We are familiar with the well-known adenoma-carcinoma sequence in the large bowel. Certainly we may postulate such a sequence for the stomach, but nevertheless: (a) Adenoma of the stomach is extremely rare. (b) Carcinogenesis is more manifold

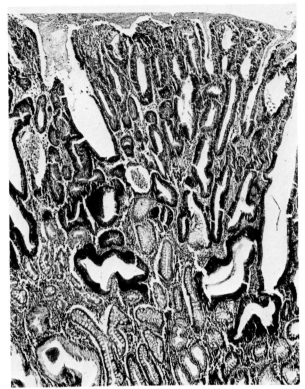

Figure 8-2. Biopsy from ulcer border shows dysplasia with reactive proliferation of neck glands, acute erosion at the surface, and intestinal metaplasia at the mucosa base. H&E stain. × 120.

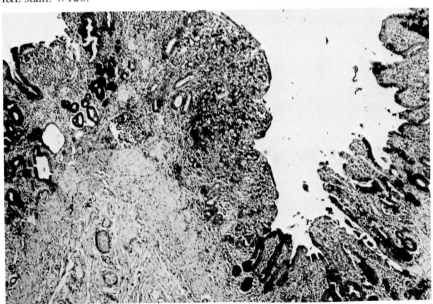

Figure 8-3. Early gastric cancer, of histologically mixed type (signet-ring cell and tubular) in part of a resected stomach. The carcinomatous growth is limited to the mucosa. H&E stain. × 40.

and complicated in the stomach. This is evident from the different histological types, as compared with only one type of adenocarcinoma of the large bowel.

RELATION OF METAPLASIA AND DYSPLASIA TO HISTOLOGICAL TYPES OF GASTRIC CANCER

Not until we have considered the different forms and types of gastric carcinoma may we draw conclusions about the early stages. It must be supposed that early cancer, seen from a histogenic standpoint, is a fully developed cancer with all the criteria for malignancy, and that every gastric cancer goes through the "early" phase. The only differences here are from a clinical aspect.

The diverse histological types may today be grouped into two basic forms, namely, in the intestinal and diffuse types of Lauren (7) and the expanding and infiltrated types of Ming (8). One may question the practical consequences of this division of histologic types.

One important difference is with respect to age at onset and the nature and frequency of an "accompanying" gastritis, as can be demonstrated in the results of our analysis of early gastric cancers (Figures 8-4 and 8-5). Thus, for example, it is irrelevant to speak only of a stom-

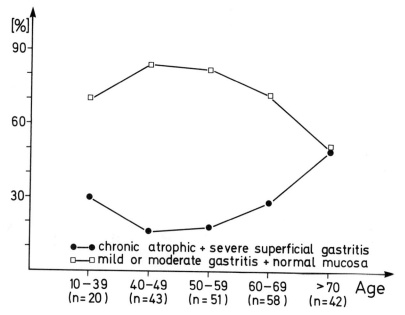

Figure 8-4.   Grades of intensity of gastritis in the fundic mucosa in relation to age in early gastric cancer (Egc) of the diffuse type.

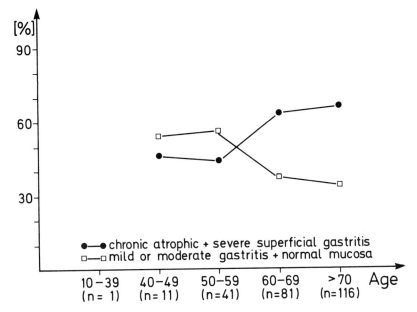

Figure 8-5.   Grades of intensity of gastritis in the fundic mucosa in relation to age in early gastric cancer (Egc) of the intestinal type.

ach cancer when one discusses, analyzes, and evaluates the findings. Without consideration of the two types, without their valuation, such findings are meaningless (9–14). The two types should especially be taken into consideration when one is searching for the so-called pre-cancers. The terms and concepts of our topics would be suitable for only about one-half of all stomach cancers even if we wanted to use them in some form of sequence. This is evident from the way we have presented our early gastric cancers, with the separation of the intestinal and diffuse types (Figure 8-6). Even if we agree with the present general concept that intestinal metaplasia and chronic atrophic gastritis pave the way for the intestinal type of carcinoma, we have shown in our studies of early gastric cancer and gastritis that this is not true for the diffuse carcinoma. We are also undecided as to whether this idea should be questioned for intestinal carcinoma as well (1, 4).

One must at least take into consideration that intestinal metaplasia not only, as mentioned before, can be a normal finding in border areas, but that dysplasia and intestinal metaplasia as well are substrates of reactive and regenerative processes. This is true not only of benign ulcers but also of carcinomas. With these facts in mind, we find that the terms "dysplasia" and "intestinal metaplasia" are superfluous for diagnostic purposes and are obsolete because they are misleading.

Typing

Intestinal	53%
Diffuse	43%
Mixed	4%

Figure 8-6.   Frequency of the different histological types in 500 cases of early gastric cancer.

DIFFICULTIES ENCOUNTERED IN APPLYING DYSPLASIA TO BIOPSY SPECIMENS

The reasons for the difficulties in the integration of dysplasia grades into practical biopsy diagnoses are as follows: The material used for dysplasia gradations was obtained primarily from resected stomachs. Thus, there are criteria that cannot always be suitably used for material that has been collected by biopsy during gastroscopy, for example, Nagayo's reference to cysts in the base of the mucosa (15). Also, the grading of dysplasia was done without respect to the age of the patients or to the localization and the nature of the basic illness, for example, erosions, ulcerations, polypoid formations, etc. Practice has taught us that cellular and structural changes, the criteria for dysplasia, are dependent on the general and the local situation and may thus be evaluated quite differently. This is the reason that we refuse to grade a dysplasia blindly, without information about clinical data and the local findings. This abstract dysplasia grading is clinically irrelevant when, for example, advice is given to "follow up," yet there is no corresponding endoscopic finding describing the localization of the dysplasia.

Concerning the results of the use of the concept of dysplasia in biopsy findings of pathologists, there are, in our opinion, two facts that are not at all positive. In pathological reports, grades of dysplasia are mentioned whether or not there is some special feature and even if the clinician is perhaps just asking about gastritis. One gets the impression that the pathologist thinks that if dysplasia is mentioned, a relevant diagnosis does not have to be given! Also, dysplasia is falsely interpreted and is mixed in with other terms dealing with precancer, so that the clinician is not only confused but may also be misled to initiate incorrect therapeutic measures.

The effects of dysplasia diagnoses on the clinician and the patient have thus been demonstrated. Such misleading conclusions derived from dysplasia findings may lead to follow-ups that may be, as we have already suggested, irrelevant if there are problems in localizing the lesion or if there is no corresponding endoscopic finding. Such endless and useless follow-ups are inconvenient for the clinician, the patient, and the wallet. At worst, they may lead to incorrect intervention.

PRECURSORS OF GASTRIC CANCER

After these negative views regarding these customary concepts, the following question might be justifiably asked: What is left as a possible precursor of stomach cancer? First: chronic atrophic gastritis with and without intestinal metaplasia in the syndrome of pernicious anemia; second: a severe dysplasia, which we designate as glandular neck proliferation with cellular atypia, or borderline lesion of the protruded type, or flat adenoma according to Ming (16; Figure 8-7); third: severe dysplasia, such as the rare adenoma of the gastric mucosa (Figure 8-8).

This is true only for gastric cancer of the intestinal type (with some reservations for the stomach in pernicious anemia). For the diffuse type, that is, for the signet-ring cell carcinoma, we know, up to now, of no precursor, except perhaps in two cases in which we found

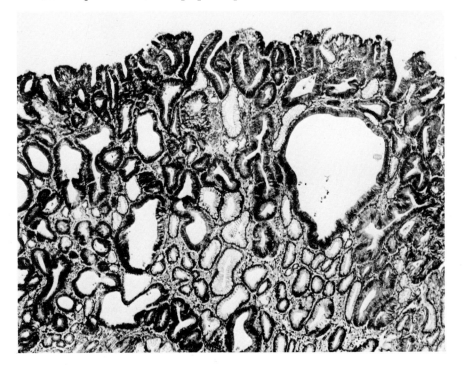

Figure 8-7. Snare biopsy of a small gastric polyp shows a borderline lesion with glandular neck cell proliferation and severe cellular atypia. H&E stain. × 120.

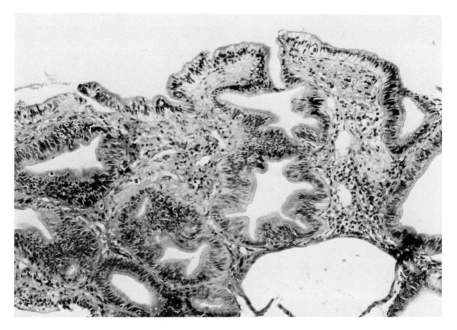

Figure 8-8.   Biopsy particle of a gastric polyp shows the superficial part of a "real" adenoma of the stomach. Glands are deformed and cystically dilated with "atypical" epithelium. An initial villous structure is also seen. H&E stain. × 150.

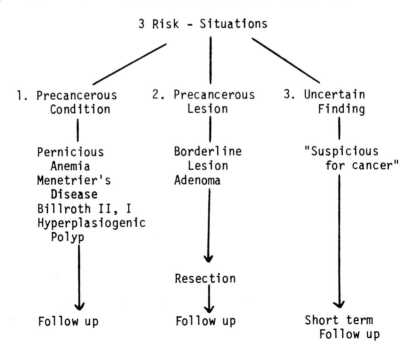

Figure 8-9.   Plan of action for the early diagnosis of gastric carcinoma.

a row of indifferent cells where there was an otherwise basic structure of the glandular body and superficial strata.

Regarding the concept of early gastric cancer, namely, the possibility of early diagnosis, if the morphologically-histologically tangible precursors are so much in question, as we have shown, then another way must be found. Our concept, which includes a plan of action for the early diagnosis of gastric cancer, is demonstrated in Figure 8-9. Since it has been possible for us to diagnose 532 early gastric cancers in the last 13 years, it can be said that this concept has proven itself. On the other hand, with a classification according to the grades of dysplasia, neither pathologist, clinician, nor the patient is helped.

REFERENCES

1. Heilmann, K. L. *Gastritis, intestinale Metaplasie, Carcinom*. Stuttgart: Thieme, 1978.
2. Grundmann, E., and Schlake, W. Histology of possible precancerous stages in stomach. In *Gastric Cancer*, edited by Herfarth, Ch., and Schlag, P., pp. 72–82. Berlin: Springer-Verlag, 1979.
3. Morson, B. C., Sobin, L. H., Grundmann, E., Johansen, A., Nagayo, T., and Serck-Hanssen, A. Precancerous conditions and epithelial dysplasia in the stomach. *J. Clin. Pathol.* 33 (1980):711–721.
4. Oehlert, W. Biological significance of dysplasia of the epithelium and of atrophic gastritis. In *Gastric Cancer*, edited by Herfarth, Ch., and Schlag, P., pp. 91–104. Berlin: Springer-Verlag, 1979.
5. Oehlert, W., Keller, P., Henke, M., and Strauch, M. Gastric mucosal dysplasia: What is its clinical significance? *Front. Gastrointest. Res.* 4 (1979):173–182.
6. Kraus, B., and Cain, H. Is there a carcinoma in-situ of gastric mucosa? *Pathol. Res. Pract.* 164 (1979):342–355.
7. Lauren, P. The two histological main types of gastric carcinoma: Diffuse and so-called intestinal-type carcinoma. *Acta Pathol. Microbiol. Scand.* 64 (1965):31–49.
8. Ming, S.-C. Gastric carcinoma. A pathobiological classification. *Cancer* 39 (1977):2475–2485.
9. Elster, K., and Thomasko, A. Klinische Wertung der histologischen Typen des Magenfrühkarzinoms. Eine Analyse von 300 Fällen. *Leber Magen Darm* 8 (1978):319–327.
10. Elster, K. Die Bedeutung der Gastritis für die Entstehung des Geschwürs und des Karzinoms. In *Speiseröhre—Magen*, edited by Boecker, W., pp. 47–52. Stuttgart: Thieme, 1979.
11. Elster, K., and Seifert, E. Magenfrühkarzinom. In *Das Gastroenterologische Kompendium, Vol. 7*, edited by Gheorghiu, Th., pp. 1–76. Baden-Baden: Witzstrock, 1979.
12. Elster, K., Thomasko, A., and Wild, A. Klinisch relevante pathologisch-anatomische Befunde an 300 Magenfrühkarzinomen. In *Das Magenkarzinom*, edited by Beger, H. G., Bergemann, W., and Oshima, H., pp. 73–79. Stuttgart: Thieme, 1980.

13. Elster, K. Das Risiko des Magenkarzinoms. In *Fortschritte der gastro-enterologischen Endoskopie, Vol. 12*, edited by Henning, H., pp. 25–28. Gräfelfing: Demeter, 1982.
14. Rösch, W., and Elster, K. Gastrointestinale Präkanzerosen. In *Das Gastroenterologische Kompendium, Vol. 1*, edited by Gheorghiu, Th., pp. 1–96. Baden-Baden: Witzstrock, 1977.
15. Nagayo, T. Dysplasia of the gastric mucosa and its relation to the precancerous state. *Gann* 72 (1981):813–823.
16. Ming, S. -C. The classification and significance of gastric polyps. In *The Gastrointestinal Tract*, edited by Yardley, J. H., and Morson, D. M., pp. 149–175. Baltimore: Williams & Wilkins, 1977.

III CHRONIC GASTRITIS

9 CHRONIC GASTRITIS AND GASTRIC CANCER

P. Correa

It is now well recognized that invasive gastric cancer is preceded by a prolonged process of progressive histologic lesions of the gastric mucosa. One of the key events in this process is chronic gastritis. There is, however, considerable heterogeneity in chronic gastritis, and not all of its variants carry an increased risk for gastric cancer. This chapter explores the clinical and pathologic features of chronic gastritis and attempts to examine their possible connection with gastric cancer.

The gastric mucosa is a specialized organ frequently exposed to injurious agents of several kinds. These agents are mostly neutralized, controlled, or partially blocked by normal defense and repair mechanisms: the mucus barrier and the regenerative capacity of the mucosa. Acute gastritis, representing recent injury, is a common finding at endoscopic examinations as well as in biopsy and autopsy material. It is nonspecific in its morphology and can be regarded as a failure of the mucosa to respond adequately to repeated acute injuries. Chronic gastritis is usually preceded by repeated bouts of acute gastritis.

Most descriptions of chronic gastritis are based on experience with specific populations. There is, however, considerable variation in the pattern of gastritis observed in different populations, probably reflecting differences in genetic and environmental factors.

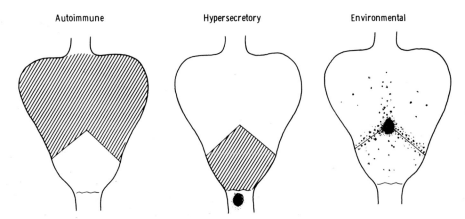

Figure 9-1.   Schematic representation of three types of chronic gastritis. The shaded areas and dark spots represent the areas involved by gastritis. The typical localization of peptic ulcers in each type of gastritis is shown.

There are many etiopathogenic entities whose morphologic substratum is a chronic inflammation of the gastric mucosa. Some of them are poorly understood and rather rare, such as Menetrier's disease, Crohn's disease, and eosinophilic gastritis. Our discussion is limited to the types that constitute frequent and important medical problems throughout the world. Although the causation of chronic gastritis is most probably multifactorial, the main types—autoimmune chronic gastritis (ACG), hypersecretory chronic gastritis (HCG), and environmental (or dietary) chronic gastritis (ECG) (1; Figure 9-1)—have one predominant etiologic factor that has been used as an identifier.

AUTOIMMUNE CHRONIC GASTRITIS

ACG is part of the pernicious anemia syndrome and has been referred to as type A gastritis (2–4). Complete gastric atrophy, the end result of chronic atrophic gastritis, has been recognized as a classic component of pernicious anemia for many years. Gastric biopsies in patients with pernicious anemia have shown complete atrophy in less than one-half of the cases; chronic atrophic gastritis and intestinal metaplasia are observed in the majority of cases (5). The lesions characteristically involve the corpus and fundus of the stomach diffusely, leaving the antrum intact (Figure 9-1). This characteristic distribution is explained by the pathogenesis of the gastric lesions: injury by autoantibodies against intrinsic factor and parietal cells. The gastrin-secreting G cells (antrally located) are also spared, and their response to hypochlorhydria, a consequence of parietal cells loss, is hyperfunction and hyperplasia resulting in hypergastrinemia. ACG increases in prevalence and severity with age and is more frequent in males than in females. Not all patients with this type of gastritis have overt pernicious anemia, but a significant proportion of them will eventually develop the syndrome. The disease is most frequently observed in populations of northern European descent. Intestinal metaplasia is a frequent sequela of ACG. The role of intestinal metaplasia as a cancer precursor is discussed in other chapters. Gastric carcinomas arising in this type of background are usually of the intestinal type.

The exact mechanism of genetic transmission of pernicious anemia is still unclear. The tendency to form gastric antibodies may be transmitted in an autosomal dominant gene with incomplete penetrance (6). Some members of such families do not have clinical manifestations of gastritis, but are found to carry parietal cell antibodies in their blood. Only with increasing age do more members of such families have overt signs of gastritis.

Intestinal metaplasia commonly accompanies ACG. Since metaplasia is positively associated with gastric cancer risk and is subject to dysplastic transformation, ACG carries a high risk for the development of gastric carcinoma with advancing age. Gastric carcinomas arising in this mucosal background are of the "intestinal" histologic type and are characteristically located in the corpus.

HYPERSECRETORY CHRONIC GASTRITIS

Peptic ulcer may be defined as a loss of integrity of the mucosa owing to acid-pepsin digestion. This definition may be useful, but it hides the fact that there are at least two etiologic entities that can lead to peptic ulcer: HCG (which could also be called psychosomatic or neurogenic gastritis) and ECG. Ulceration is only a temporary manifestation of the pathologic process, and it is unfortunate that it has been chosen as the cornerstone of clinical classification. From the etiologic point of view, a clinical diagnosis of peptic ulcer is incomplete and should be followed by a characterization of the type of gastritis present: HCG or ECG. Much of the controversy surrounding the ulcer-cancer relationship is due to a lack of recognition of the two etiologic entities. The need to individualize them is more than Byzantine, since they have markedly different natural histories. For all practical purposes, duodenal ulcers form part of the HCG syndrome. Gastric ulcers, although mostly "peptic" by definition, may form part of either HCG or ECG complexes. It may sometimes be hard to decide which etiology is determining the presence of an ulcer in a given individual, and there is reason to believe that both etiologic entities may coexist in some patients. In their pure form, however, both types of gastritis have precise morphologic characteristics that may help clinicians decide which is responsible for the syndrome in any given patient.

One of the most characteristic features of HCG is its topographic localization. If the ulcer is duodenal, the chronic gastritis is limited to the antrum; the corpus and fundus remain morphologically normal or show minimal focal acute superficial gastritis (7). When the ulcer accompanying the HCG complex is localized in the stomach, the gastritis is present in the antrum but may also extend to the corpus. This extension is determined by the localization of the ulcer: In prepyloric ulcers 76 percent of the patients have normal fundal mucosa, compared with 26 percent in angulus ulcers and 7 percent in midcorpus ulcers (8). The corpus gastritis observed in such cases is present in the immediate vicinity of the ulcer and could be interpreted as part of the

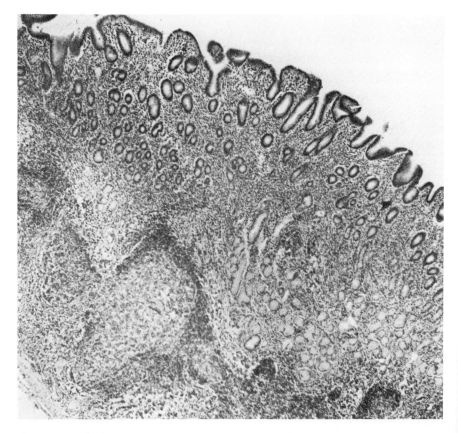

Figure 9-2.   Chronic (hypersecretory) gastritis associated with duodenal peptic ulcer. There is marked lymphocytic infiltration, with the presence of lymphoid follicles and no atrophy. H&E stain. × 50.

inflammatory process responding to tissue necrosis. The ulcer itself is usually in the antral side of the corpus-antrum junction line (2). It should be remembered that the lesser curvature has antral-type glands. The gross morphology just described is very different from what is observed in ECG, as will be described later.

Histologically, HCG is characterized by hyperplasia of the surface epithelium, resulting in elongation of the suprafoveolar folds, frequently with less than normal amounts of mucus in the cytoplasm, and by marked lymphocytic infiltration of the lamina propria, usually with lymphoid follicles and germinal centers (Figures 9-2 and 9-3). Antral gastritis precedes duodenal ulcers.

When HCG leads to gastric ulcers, they tend to be immediately adjacent or very close to the pylorus (7). Atrophy of glands may be present but is not a prominent feature. Intestinal metaplasia is absent in most cases and when present tends to be of mild degree. The ulcer itself is not located in the midst of an area of intestinal metaplasia. The excessive representation of patients with blood group A observed in ACG is not observed in HCG.

Excessive secretion of hydrochloric acid and pepsin is found in HCG. It has been postulated that the secretion is so excessive that the normal mucus production of the epithelial cells becomes inadequate to protect the mucosa from the repeated injury. When this happens, the gastric juice ulcerates the mucosa by a process of digestion (9). The weakest point would be determined by the degree of loss of mucus protection and the excessive exposure to acid and pepsin. This often occurs in that part of the duodenal mucosa directly facing the jet of gastric secretion or in the gastric mucosa in the immediate vicinity of the pyloric sphincter where hyperacid gastric juice is detained.

In spite of excessive gastric acid-pepsin secretion, gastrin blood levels are elevated and gastrin activity per gram of antral mucosa is increased in patients with HCG. This represents an apparent failure of the feedback mechanism, which must be related somehow to whatever is the cause of this syndrome, presumably abnormal psychogenic or neurogenic stimuli transmitted via the autonomic nervous system.

ENVIRONMENTAL CHRONIC GASTRITIS

ECG is part of a complex of lesions usually covered under the term "gastritis type B" (3). It is prevalent in certain parts of the world, especially eastern and northern Europe, the U.S.S.R., Japan, and the Andean parts of South and Central America. Its geographic distribution coincides with the areas of high gastric cancer risk (of the so-called

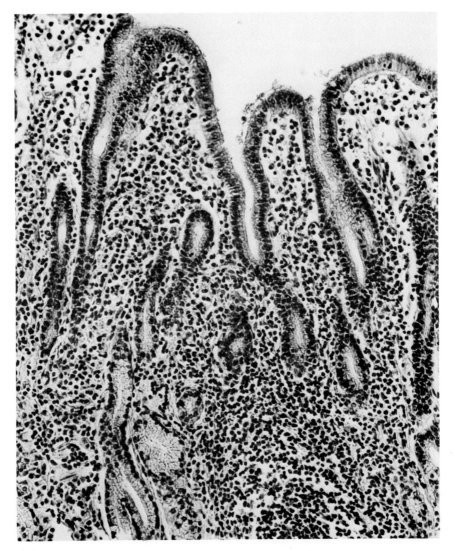

Figure 9-3.   Chronic (hypersecretory) gastritis associated with peptic ulcer of the duodenum. Note the marked lymphoid infiltration and elongation of the suprafoveolar portion of the mucosa to form pseudovilli. H&E stain. × 250.

epidemic or intestinal type) (10–12). It has been slowly realized that the two syndromes ECG and carcinoma are part of the same etiologic complex (13). Studies of populations at high gastric cancer risk in different parts of the world have focused on the role of chronic gastritis as the gastric cancer precursor (14). The first evidence of injury of the gastric mucosa begins early in life, usually around the second decade. By the age of 20 to 25 years, the individuals in a community who will develop chronic gastritis already have histologic indications of the beginning of the process. In populations where gastric cancer is infrequent, the proportion of chronic gastritis is usually less than 20 percent, whereas in high-risk populations that proportion is usually 70 percent or higher. At the early stages the clinical manifestations of gastritis are vague or nonexistent. Population surveys have found no correlations between symptoms and histologic changes at this stage (12, 14). With more advanced gastritis, postprandial epigastric heaviness, pyrosis, sour taste, nausea, and vomitus have been described. Later on, some patients develop gastric peptic ulcer, usually treated medically and occasionally surgically. In spite of treatment or the lack of it, the ulcer later heals and the patient enters slowly into the gastric atrophy-hypochlorhydria-achlorhydria syndrome. A number of patients with this symptom complex develop gastric carcinoma, usually without reaching a complete achlorhydric status.

The distribution of ECG lesions in the gastric mucosa is very characteristic (Figure 9-1). It is basically multifocal and involves the antrum as well as the corpus. In its early stages, multiple small foci appear along the corpus-antrum junction line and spread as new small foci appear in the lesser curvature above and below the junction. Each

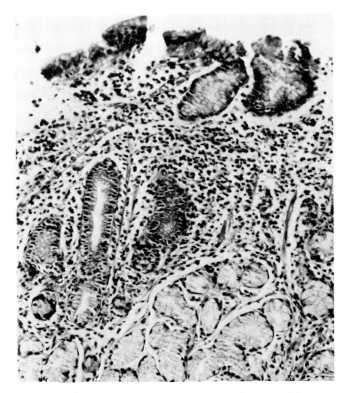

Figure 9-4.   Superficial gastritis. Mononuclear cell infiltration of the upper portion of the mucosa and hyperplasia of the glandular necks are seen. H&E stain. × 180.

focus then grows, covers a larger surface area, and becomes confluent with neighboring foci to involve larger and larger areas in both the antrum and the corpus and finally the fundus. The dynamics of this extension have been inferred from detailed topographic analyses of histologic sections of autopsy material. Autopsy specimens from younger individuals show the presumably early foci to be located around the corpus-antrum junction line, whereas similar specimens from older individuals show larger foci and confluence (10). The same conclusions are reached when surgical specimens are stained grossly for intestinal-type enzymes (alkaline phosphatase, sucrase, leucine aminopeptidase), which appear as a consequence of the metaplastic process (15).

Histologically, ECG includes many changes that apparently form a continuum. Several stages may be present in different areas of the mucosa, but not all lesions are observed in any one stomach. In our experience the spectrum of lesions can be divided into the following stages: superficial gastritis (SG), atrophic gastritis, intestinal metaplasia, and dysplasia. The last stage is not reached by most of the patients

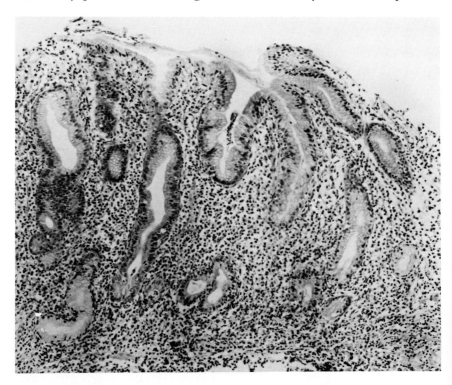

Figure 9-5.   Chronic atrophic gastritis. The loss of glands results in extensive areas of the lamina propria occupied by inflammatory infiltrate. Glandular neck hyperplasia is present. H&E stain. × 125.

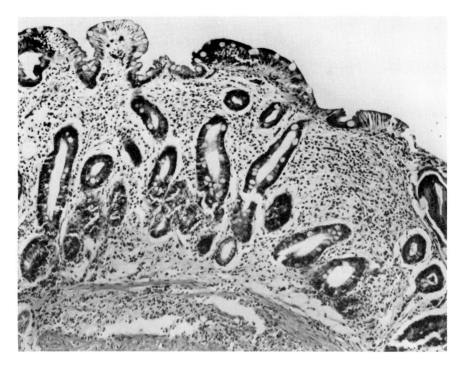

Figure 9-6.   Chronic atrophic gastritis with extensive intestinal metaplasia of the glands and the surface epithelium. H&E stain. × 125.

and is very close to the final stages of malignant transformation. SG (Figure 9-4) is characterized by a chronic inflammatory infiltrate limited to the most superficial portion of the lamina propria and hyperplasia of the glandular necks. It may also show polynuclear infiltration of the epithelium of the glandular necks. The next more serious lesion represents atrophic changes and is recognizable because extensive areas of the lamina propria are devoid of glands (Figure 9-5). In this stage the chronic infiltration and the neck hyperplasia are usually still present in variable degrees of severity. On this background the next step is seen when metaplastic glands appear to replace the original glands lost during the process of atrophy (Figure 9-6).

Intestinal metaplasia and its heterogeneity are discussed in other chapters. In our experience the dysplastic lesions are observed mostly on the background of atrophy and metaplasia, but there seem to be considerable differences among populations, apparently reflecting exposures to different mixes of etiologic factors. In Colombia, where the predominant factors are low intake of animal proteins and high intake of salt, nitrates, and fava beans (16), most of the dysplastic lesions are of the adenomatous type (Type I) (17, 18; Figure 9-7). These are usually associated with well-differentiated adenocarcinomas of

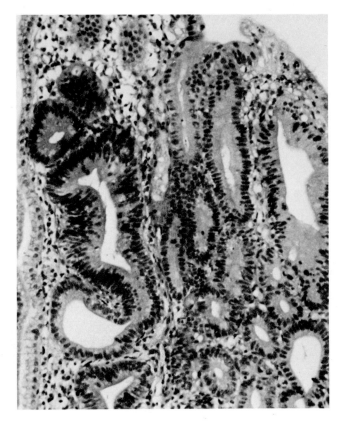

Figure 9-7.   Adenomatous dysplasia. Note the back-to-back tubules lined by elongated, crowded, hyperchromatic nuclei. H&E stain. × 180.

the intestinal type. In New Orleans, although the same basic process is seen, the inflammatory component is more prominent, and the hyperplastic (Type II) dysplasias are more frequent (Figure 9-8). They are also associated with intestinal-type carcinomas, but they tend to be less differentiated, as described by Jass (18). The etiologic factors in New Orleans are not yet well identified, but the disease is observed predominantly in blacks and it is suspected that certain alcoholic beverages may play a role.

MICROENVIRONMENT

There is a complex interrelationship between the mucosal lesions and the gastric content. Some unknown dietary factor or factors induce chronic gastritis; atrophic gastritis leads to higher pH in the gastric cavity, which leads to bacterial growth; bacteria reduce dietary nitrate to nitrite; and nitrite is capable of reacting with nitrogen-containing

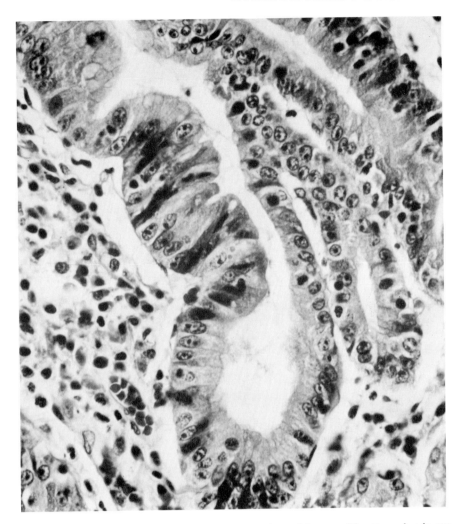

Figure 9-8. Hyperplastic dysplasia. Tortuous, branching proliferative glands are present, along with nuclear irregularity and pseudostratification. H&E stain. ×325.

substances (ingested food, drugs, or regurgitated bile) to form N-nitroso compounds, many of which are mutagenic and possibly carcinogenic. This chain of events, therefore, perpetuates injury to the gastric mucosa and potentially induces more advanced dysplastic lesions and eventually carcinoma (19).

REFERENCES

1. Correa, P. The epidemiology and pathogenesis of chronic gastritis: Three etiologic entities. *Front. Gastroenterol. Res.* 6 (1980):98–108.
2. Lambert, R. Chronic gastritis. *Digestion* 7 (1972):83–126.

3. Strickland, R. G., and Mackay, I. R. A reappraisal of the nature and significance of chronic atrophic gastritis. *Am. J. Dig. Dis.* 18(1973):426–440.
4. Chatterjee, D. Idiopathic chronic gastritis. *Surg. Gynecol. Obstet.* 143 (1976): 986–1000.
5. Joske, R. A., Finckh, E. S., and Wood, I. G. Gastric biopsies. *Q. J. Med.* 24 (1955):269–294.
6. Wangel, A. G., Callender, S. T., Spray, G. H., and Wright, R. A family study of pernicious anemia. *Br. J. Haematol.* 14 (1968):183–204.
7. Stemmermann, G., Haenszel, W., and Locke, F. Epidemiologic pathology of gastric ulcer and gastric carcinoma among Japanese in Hawaii. *J. Natl. Cancer Inst.* 58 (1977):13–20.
8. Stadelmann, O., Elster, K., Stolte, M., Miederer, S. F., Deyhle, P., Demling, L., and Siegenthaler, W. The peptic gastric ulcer. Histotopographic and functional investigations. *Scand. J. Gastroenterol.* 6 (1971):613–623.
9. Sun, D. C. H. Etiology and pathology of peptic ulcer. In *Gastroenterology,* 3rd ed., edited by Bockus, H. L., pp. 579–610. Philadelphia: W. B. Saunders, 1974.
10. Correa, P., Cuello, C., and Duque, E. Carcinoma and intestinal metaplasia of the stomach in Colombian migrants. *J. Natl. Cancer Inst.* 44 (1970):297–306.
11. Imai, T., Kubo, T., and Watanabe, H. Chronic gastritis in Japanese with reference to high incidence of gastric carcinoma. *J. Natl. Cancer Inst.* 47 (1971):179–195.
12. Siurala, M., Isokoski, M., and Varis, K. Prevalence of gastritis in a rural population. *Scand. J. Gastroenterol.* 3 (1968):211–223.
13. Correa, P. Precursors of gastric and esophageal cancer. *Cancer* 50 (1982): 2445–2565.
14. Correa, P., Cuello, C., Duque, E., Burbano, L., Garcia, F. T., Bolanos, O., Brown, C., and Haenszel, W. Gastric cancer in Colombia. III. The natural history of precursor lesions. *J. Natl. Cancer Inst.* 57 (1976):1027–1035.
15. Stemmermann, G., and Hayashi, T. Intestinal metaplasia of the gastric mucosa: A gross and microscopic study of its distribution in various disease states. *J. Natl. Cancer Inst.* 41 (1968):627–634.
16. Correa, P., Cuello, C., Fajardo, F., Haenszel, W., Bolanos, O., and de Ramirez, B. Diet and gastric cancer: Nutrition survey in a high risk area. *J. Natl. Cancer Inst.* 70 (1983):673–678.
17. Cuello, C., Correa, P., Zarama, G., Lopez, J., Murray, J., and Gordillo, G. Histopathology of gastric dysplasia. *Am. J. Surg. Pathol.* 3 (1979):491–500.
18. Jass, J. R. A classification of gastric dysplasia. *Histopathology* 7 (1983):181–183.
19. Correa, P. The gastric precancerous process. *Cancer Surveys.* 1984 (in press).

10 CHRONIC GASTRITIS: A DYNAMIC PROCESS TOWARD CANCER?

R. Cheli, A. Giacosa, and A. Perasso

The histobioptic experience has demonstrated for a long time that chronic gastritis is fundamentally expressed by two main aspects: an early one characterized by the presence of inflammatory phenomena in the superficial layer of the mucosa, and a late one in which the inflammatory phenomena extend to the deep portion of the mucosa with marked reduction of the glandular component. Since the first descriptions of Schindler (1), these two patterns have been defined as superficial gastritis and atrophic gastritis.

The possible evolution from superficial to atrophic gastritis is supported by multiple data. First, bioptic study has clearly shown the existence of intermediate phases of the process: In our experience, the superficial and atrophic steps are interposed by a preatrophic phase characterized by an expansion of the superficial inflammatory infiltrates and a partial reduction of the glandular parenchyma. Other terms for preatrophic gastritis are "gastric subatrophy" and "partial atrophy." The time required for the evolution from superficial to atrophic gastritis has been evaluated by Siurala et al. (2). These authors demonstrated by means of stochastic analysis that the progression requires about 19 years. Another point concerns the prevalence of atrophic lesions in patients over 50 years of age (3). Beside these findings a further anatomicopathological pattern may be observed, even though rarely—that of follicular gastritis, which is characterized by hyperplasia of the lymphofollicles.

Later, Whitehead (4) introduced the concept of "activity" in the classification criteria of chronic gastritis, correlating this terminology with the presence of neutrophils in the inflammatory infiltrate as an expression of acute phenomena. This finding is of importance because it indicates the overlap of acute inflammation on a chronic condition that is not modified as far as its fundamental histological features are concerned.

More recently, the introduction of cell count techniques has been very important (5). This method has revealed the increase of lymphocytes within the surface epithelium and of plasmacytes and lymphocytes in the lamina propria in chronic gastritis. Moreover, the quantitative evaluation of parietal cells has demonstrated their progressive reduction during the evolution toward the atrophic stage.

HISTOLOGICAL CLASSIFICATION OF CHRONIC GASTRITIS

The classification of chronic gastritis is not easy since the standardization of the different patterns is in contrast with the evolutionary character of the disease process. As previously mentioned, the different extension of the inflammatory state and the variable entity of glandular damage lead to the definition of four fundamental patterns of chronic gastritis: superficial gastritis, preatrophic gastritis, atrophic gastritis, and follicular gastritis (6). From this classification we excluded the so-called gastric atrophy, since the term "gastric atrophy" is not morphologically correct, it being impossible to differentiate this condition from atrophic gastritis (7).

Considering the variability of the gastric mucosa, the distribution of the inflammatory lesions, and the scarce material obtained by a forceps biopsy, some rules have to be respected. We suggest that at least six endoscopic biopsies be taken in each case: four in the gastric body, immediately above the angulus (lesser curvature, greater curvature, anterior and posterior wall), and two in the antrum, within 3 centimeters of the pylorus (anterior and posterior wall) (8).

Superficial gastritis is the most frequent condition. In it the thickness of the fundic mucosa ranges from 0.8 to 1.2 millimeters, as in normal mucosa. The cells of the surface epithelium show variable diameter and frequently are interrupted by microerosions. Within the epithelium there is an increased number of lymphocytes, which are

Table 10-1. Lymphocyte Count in the Surface Epithelium
in Chronic Gastritis.

Conditions	No. of Cases	Surface Epithelium (lymphocytes/mm)
Controls	19	8.1 ± 2.3
Superficial gastritis	33	33.6 ± 7.2 ($p < 0.001$)
Preatrophic gastritis	21	57.4 ± 12.4 ($p < 0.001$)
Atrophic gastritis	18	66.8 ± 14.7 ($p < 0.001$)
Follicular gastritis	6	25.7 ± 3.4 ($p < 0.001$)

Source: Giacosa et al. (5).

irregularly distributed (Tables 10-1 and 10-2). The foveolae are elongated and deformed. In the interfoveolar area, a rich inflammatory cell population constituted by plasmacytes and lymphocytes is constantly observed (Figure 10-1). In some interfoveolar areas, reticular fibers form a thick stroma. In 50 percent of cases the reticular thickness also involves the interglandular region, even though in all cases glandular tubuli are normal, with slight degenerative phenomena localized in the neck area.

Preatrophic gastritis represents a transitional condition between superficial and atrophic gastritis. The mucosal thickness ranges from 0.4 to 0.6 millimeters and is strictly correlated with the degree of glandular reduction. The surface epithelium consists of vacuolar cells with a high number of lymphocytes; metaplastic cells of the intestinal or goblet type may also be found. Foveolae are elongated and often tortuous. The parenchymatous component is reduced: Glandular cells show degenerative changes and often are substituted for by metaplas-

Table 10-2. Inflammatory Cell Count and Identification
in Chronic Gastritis

Conditions	No. of Cases	Plasmacytes	Lymphocytes	Other Cells	Total
Controls	19	1,616 ± 379	1,460 ± 378	1,358 ± 315	4,434 ± 465
Superficial gastritis	33	4,408 ± 682 ($p < 0.001$)	1,538 ± 386 (NS)	1,660 ± 335 (NS)	7,606 ± 450 ($p < 0.001$)
Preatrophic gastritis	21	6,570 ± 608 ($p < 0.001$)	1,871 ± 546 (NS)	1,697 ± 432 (NS)	10,138 ± 520 ($p < 0.001$)
Atrophic gastritis	18	6,320 ± 495 ($p < 0.001$)	1,683 ± 417 (NS)	1,430 ± 381 (NS)	9,433 ± 603 ($p < 0.001$)
Follicular gastritis	6	—	23,550 ± 1,141 ($p < 0.001$)	—	23,550 ± 1,141 ($p < 0.001$)

Values are expressed as cells/mm³.
Source: Giacosa et al. (5).

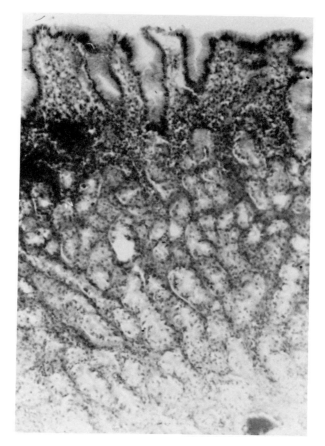

Figure 10-1.   Superficial gastritis of the fundic mucosa. H&E stain. × 108.

tic cells. The parietal cells are diminished. The interglandular connective tissue is rich in inflammatory cells (Figure 10-2; Tables 10-1 and 10-2), which extend to the muscularis mucosae. The inter- and perglandular fibers are thickened and occasionally transformed into collagenous tissue.

In atrophic gastritis the mucosa thickness is less than 0.5 millimeter. The surface epithelium is cubic, reduced in height, and frequently interrupted by erosions (Figure 10-3). Metaplastic cells, constituted by goblet or enterocyte-like cells with brush borders, are common. The lymphocyte count within the surface epithelium shows a marked increase in comparison with that of normal mucosa. Foveolae are usually elongated, tortuous, and occasionally fingerlike in appearance.

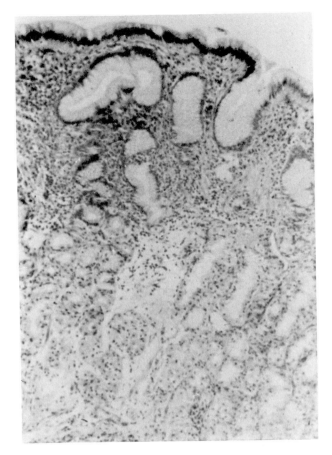

Figure 10-2.　Preatrophic gastritis of the fundic mucosa. H&E stain. × 108.

Glandular tubules are markedly reduced or have even disappeared. Among the different cell types, parietal cells are severely reduced. In the residual glandular tissue, metaplastic cells may be seen with characters similar to those described for surface epithelium. Epithelial dysplasia of the mild type (cells with slender, elongated, and hyperchromatic nuclei) is found in 10 percent of cases. Probably these findings are an expression of regenerative or hyperplastic phenomena, not representing a "true" dysplasia. The connective tissue of the lamina propria is thickened in most cases, with frequent evidence of collagenous elements. Moreover, in the stroma inflammatory cells are irregularly and diffusely distributed, with a marked increase in and

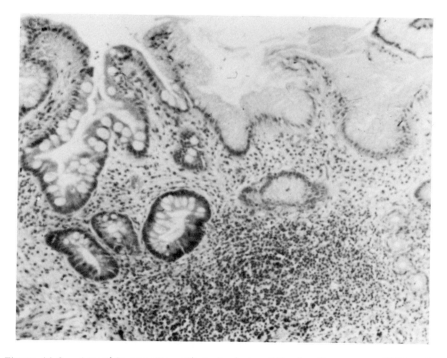

Figure 10-3.   Atrophic gastritis with metaplasia of the fundic mucosa. H&E stain.
× 108.

prevalence of plasmacytes and lymphocytes (Tables 10-1 and 10-2). The muscularis mucosae often appear hyperplastic, with degenerative phenomena, fragmentation of fibrocytes, and inflammatory cell infiltrates. In some cases the above-described phenomena are associated with hyperplasia of the superficial layer, with fingerlike protruding structures. This particular picture is generally defined as "atrophic-hyperplastic gastritis."

Follicular (or interstitial) gastritis is a rare finding (4 percent of cases) characterized by zonal inflammatory infiltrates represented mainly by lymphocytes assuming the aspect of activated lymphofollicles with a central pale zone and peripheral dark ring. These infiltrates are variably extended in the interglandular area (Figure 10-4; Tables 10-1 and 10-2).

The described alterations pertain to the fundic mucosa. In the antrum chronic gastritis has similar characteristics. The only different

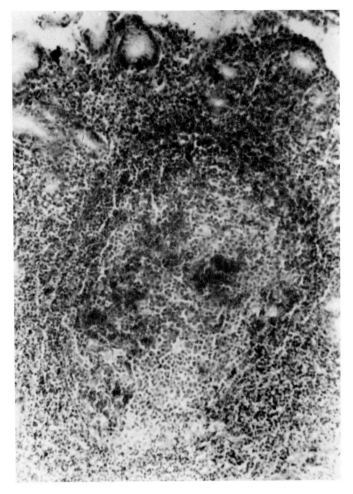

Figure 10-4. Follicular gastritis of the antral mucosa. H&E stain. × 200.

features are bestowed by the involvement of glandular elements that specifically characterize the antral parenchyma.

FUNCTIONAL BEHAVIOR OF CHRONIC GASTRITIS

The dynamic character of chronic gastritis is also confirmed by the comparison between the anatomic and functional data. Considering the fundic mucosa, in superficial gastritis the prevalent behavior is normochlorhydria, in correlation with parenchymatous normality. In preatrophic gastritis, hypochlorhydria prevails, in accordance with a parenchymatous reduction. In atrophic gastritis most of the cases show achlorhydria, which is in agreement with the great damage to the glandular component (6, 9). In follicular gastritis, our experiences have revealed the prevalence of normochlorhydria, which is in harmony with the observation of a normal parenchyma.

New contributions to this work have been obtained with simultaneous evaluation of both antral and fundic mucosa and of gastrinemia (10). These studies confirmed the correlation between HCl and parietal cell mass expressed by a "parietal index" (parietal cell count in a unit area of the tissue section). The progressive decrease of the parietal index in the entities of fundic gastritis is parallel to a marked decrease of HCl secretion with true achlorhydria when fundic atrophy is present (Table 10-3).

On the contrary, serum gastrin levels show an inverse correlation with the histological pattern of fundic mucosa and therefore also with HCl. As a matter of fact, the gastrinemic increase is high in the presence of atrophic fundic gastritis, particularly when fundic atrophy is associated with normal antral mucosa. The degree of antral damage regulates the gastrinemic increase, with even normal gastrin values when fundic atrophy is associated with antral atrophy. This behavior underscores the fact that gastrinemia does not represent a sure marker of the gastritic situation, if not considered in relation to histomorphological patterns of fundic and antral mucosa.

Morphofunctional evaluations of the gastric mucosa are needed and have to be extensive and simultaneous in order to fulfill the correct and modern concept of anatomicofunctional diagnosis of chronic gastritis.

Table 10-3. Correlation between Histological Observation, HCl Output, and Gastrinemia

| Case No. | Histology | | | HCl | Fasting Gastrinemia |
	Fundus	Antrum	Parietal Index	Maximal Acid Output (mEq/h)	(pg/ml)
13	N	N	425.3 ± 82.1	14.7 ± 9.3	65 ± 28
10	N	S + F	471.2 ± 94.7	19.2 ± 3.9	77 ± 18
12	N	A	385.0 ± 56.6	20.3 ± 2.3	70 ± 26
7	S + F	N	420.2 ± 51.3	17.4 ± 5.1	76 ± 15
6	S	S	403.2 ± 66.5	15.2 ± 5.3	82 ± 23
5	S	A	342.0 ± 73.2	17.5 + 2.1	60 ± 17
5	P	S	88.9 ± 7.0	3.2 ± 0.6	115 ± 18
4	P	A	102.4 ± 6.1	2.5 ± 1.2	76 ± 14
15	A	N	9.9 ± 0.9	0	515 ± 186
7	A	S	47.9 ± 6.6	1.2 ± 0.5	155 ± 36
5	A	A	87.0 ± 8.1	1.6 ± 0.8	80 ± 16

N, normal mucosa; S, superficial gastritis; P, preatrophic gastritis; A, atrophic gastritis; F, follicular gastritis.
Source: Giacosa et al. (10).

EPIDEMIOLOGY OF CHRONIC GASTRITIS

A constant observation coming from all bioptic experiences is related to the close correlation between atrophic gastritis and the age of patients; that is, with an increase in age, there is also an increased prevalence of chronic gastritis.

Siurala et al. (11), in a randomized histobioptic study performed in a rural Finnish population, reported the presence of chronic gastritis in 53 percent of cases and specifically of atrophic gastritis in 28 percent, with a linear increase with age. However, these authors observed that the incidence of superficial gastritis was constant. This demonstrates that a dynamic balance existed between subjects who developed a superficial gastritis and those who progressed toward atrophic gastritis.

A comparative epidemiological study of asymptomatic Italian and Hungarian subjects showed the presence of atrophic gastritis in 22 percent of the former and in 37 percent of the latter, with a progressive increase in prevalence with age in both groups (3). Similar findings were obtained when intestinal metaplasia was considered, since it occurred in 11 percent of Italians older than 60 years and in 24 percent of Hungarians of similar age, whereas for younger subjects it did not differ in the two groups (3). As previously reported, the mean time required for the evolution from superficial to atrophic gastritis is 19 years (2). These experiences were confirmed with a stochastic evaluation of the results, that is, with the transposition of cross-sectional data to longitudinal temporal data (12). Using this method it was possible to find an earlier appearance of antral gastritis in comparison with fundic gastritis and a progressive increase of inflammatory phenomena with age in both antral and fundic mucosa. Therefore, age surely represents a fundamental factor in the natural history of chronic gastritis.

CHRONIC GASTRITIS AND CANCER

In the past there were frequent reports of association between pernicious anemia and fundic atrophic gastritis and gastric cancer (13–15). Similarly, Hurst (16) and Comfort et al. (17) reported the presence of histamine-resistant achlorhydria in patients who subsequently developed gastric cancer. In 1957 Hitchcock et al. (18) indirectly confirmed this observation, demonstrating that cancer was five times more frequent in achlorhydric subjects when compared with normochlorhydric subjects.

More recently, histobioptic experiences have added new data for the correlation between atrophic gastritis and cancer. Siurala et al. (19, 20), following 116 patients with atrophic fundic gastritis for 15 years, found that 7.7 percent of the cases developed gastric cancer during the observation time. In our experience (21) a follow-up study of 363 patients 11 to 18 years after gastric biopsies and HCl secretion test revealed the development of gastric carcinoma in 13 percent of 65 cases with prior finding of atrophic gastritis. In the study of Siurala et al. (20), the mean interval time between initial biopsy and gastric cancer diagnosis was 15 years, whereas in our study it was 8 years. Findley et al. (22), following a group of 100 patients with atrophic gastritis, did not observe gastric cancer in any of the cases reexamined within a 5-year period. However, it remains undetermined how long the gastritis process had existed in these patients before their first examination.

In these reports the biological key that could explain the possible evolution from atrophic gastritis to gastric cancer is missing. Further contributions in this field come from experiences of Nieburgs and Glass (23), showing in pernicious anemia a systemic cellular maturation disorder in blood and in epithelial cells, including those of the gastric mucosa. These authors (23), reporting nuclear alterations owing to altered cellular differentiation not only in gastric tumor cells and in those of pernicious anemia but also in atrophic gastritis in the absence of anemia, hypothesized a relationship between the alterations of atrophic gastritis and gastric carcinoma.

Role of Metaplasia

In order to solve this problem, the possible role played by metaplasia was evaluated. As previously mentioned, intestinal metaplasia is almost a rule in atrophic gastritis. Morson (24) and Cheli et al. (25) showed that chronic atrophic gastritis with diffuse intestinal metaplasia is present in 90 percent of cases with gastric carcinoma. These data were afterward confirmed by immunological (26), histochemical (27), and electron microscopic studies (28).

However, it must be kept in mind that intestinal metaplasia may also be observed in the normal adult stomach although in a quantitatively minimal amount. This observation limits the specificity of the association between gastric cancer and metaplasia. Nevertheless, metaplasia is generally linked with cellular renewal as in atrophic gastritis

(29). Perhaps under these conditions cancer may be expected to develop.

Role of Dysplasia

More recently, particular interest has been given to the dysplastic phenomena associated with atrophic gastritis. In particular, Nagayo (30) hypothesized the irreversibility of severe dysplastic lesions that were potentially correlated with cancer. In our experience (31) dysplasia was rarely associated with atrophic gastritis or with metaplasia. Moreover, the degree of dysplasia was generally mild and almost always expressive of regenerative phenomena.

Therefore, it appears difficult to consider as relevant the role of dysplasia in the sequence of atrophic gastritis to cancer, and the problem remains open for further investigations.

CONCLUSIONS

Chronic gastritis is an anatomicopathological entity with a natural history characterized by a dynamic process that generally progresses from superficial inflammatory phenomena to atrophic stages. The morphological patterns have physiological correlates, so that we can consider chronic gastritis an anatomicofunctional condition.

There are still many uncertainties about the clinical meaning of chronic gastritis, since it is often symptomless and occurs occasionally with dyspepsia. At present, the state of knowledge is dominated by the epidemiologic consideration that atrophic gastritis represents a high-risk condition for cancer development. However, the link between atrophic gastritis and cancer is missing. The biological key of this evolution has been attributed previously to metaplasia, and more recently to dysplasia. However, the significance of metaplasia has been shown only by epidemiological data, and even less information is at present available regarding the role of dysplasia.

REFERENCES

1. Schindler, R. *Gastritis*. New York: Grune and Stratton, 1947.
2. Siurala, M., Varis, K., Kekki, M., and Isokoski, M. Epidemiology of gastritis. In *Modern Gastroenterology*, edited by Gregor O., and Riedl, O., pp. 540–542. Stuttgart: Schattauer Verlag, 1969.

3. Cheli, R., Simon, L., Aste, H., Figus, I. A., Nicolo, G., Bajtai, A., and Puntoni, R. Atrophic gastritis and intestinal metaplasia in asymptomatic Hungarian and Italian population. *Endoscopy* 12 (1980):105–108.

4. Whitehead, R. *Mucosal Biopsy of the Gastrointestinal Tract*. Philadelphia: W.B. Saunders, 1973.

5. Giacosa, A., Molinari, F., and Cheli, R. Analyse quantitative et qualitative des cellules inflammatoires dans les gastrites chroniques. *Acta Endosc.* 9 (1979): 105–110.

6. Cheli, R. La biopsie gastrique dans l'étude de la physiologie et de la physiopathologie de l'estomac. In *La Biopsie Gastrique par Sonde*, pp. 41–45. Paris: Masson, 1966.

7. Cheli, R., and Giacosa, A. Chronic atrophic gastritis and gastric mucosal atrophy—One and same. *Gastrointest. Endosc.* 29 (1983):23–25.

8. Cheli, R. Workshop on the histomorphology of chronic gastritis—Genova, 1982. *Ital. J. Gastroenterol.* 15 (1983):206.

9. Burhol, P. G., and Myren, J. Gastritis and gastric secretion. In *The Physiology of Gastric Secretion*, p. 626. Oslo: Universitats Vorlaget, 1968.

10. Giacosa, A., Turello, V., and Icardi, A. Sécrétion gastrique acide, gastrinémie et masse cellulaire pariétale dans les gastrites chroniques. *Gastroenterol. Clin. Biol.* 2 (1978):133–137.

11. Siurala, M. Isokoski, M., Varis, K., and Kekki, M. Prevalence of gastritis in a rural population. Bioptic study of subjects selected at random. *Scand. J. Gastroenterol.* 3 (1968):211–223.

12. Kekki, M., Ihamaki, T., Varis, K., Isokoski, M., Lehtola, J., Hovinen, E., and Siurala, M. Age of gastric cancer patients and susceptibility to chronic gastritis in their relatives. A mathematical approach using Poisson's process and scoring of gastritis state. *Scand. J. Gastroenterol.* 8 (1973):673–679.

13. Jenner, A. W. F. Perniziose anämie und Magenkarzinom. *Acta Med. Scand.* 102 (1939):529–534.

14. Riegler, R. G., and Kaplan, H. S. Pernicious anemia and the early diagnosis of tumors of the stomach. *JAMA* 128 (1945): 426–432.

15. Magnus, H. A. A reassessment of gastric lesions in pernicious anaemia. *J. Clin. Pathol.* 11 (1958):289–294.

16. Hurst, A. F. On the precursor of carcinoma of the stomach. *Lancet* 217 (1929):1023–1027.

17. Comfort, M. W., Butsch, W. L., and Eustermann, G. B. Observations on gastric acidity before and after development of carcinoma of the stomach. *Am. J. Dig. Dis.* 4 (1937):673–679.

18. Hitchcock, C. R., McLean, L. D., and Sullivan, W. A. The secretory and clinical aspects of achlorhydria and gastric atrophy as precursor of gastric cancer. *J. Natl. Cancer Inst.* 18 (1957):795–801.

19. Siurala, M., and Seppala, K. Atrophic gastritis as a possible precursor of gastric carcinoma and pernicious anemia. *Acta Med. Scand.* 166 (1960):455–461.

20. Siurala, M., Varis, K., and Wiljasalo, M. Studies of patients with atrophic gastritis: A 10–15 year follow-up. *Scand. J. Gastroenterol.* 1 (1966):40–48.

21. Cheli, R., Santi, L., Ciancamerla, G., and Canciani, G. A clinical and statistical follow-up study of atrophic gastritis. *Am. J. Dig. Dis.* 18 (1973):1061–1066.

22. Findley, J. W., Kirsner, J. B., and Palmer, W. L. Atrophic gastritis: A follow-up study of 100 patients. *Gastroenterology* 16 (1950):347–351.

23. Nieburgs, H. E., and Glass, G. B. J. Gastric cell maturation disorders in atrophic gastritis, pernicious anemia and carcinoma. *Am. J. Dig. Dis.* 8 (1963):135–159.
24. Morson, B. C. Intestinal metaplasia of the gastric mucosa. *Br. J. Cancer* 9 (1955):365–376.
25. Cheli, R., Dodero, M., and Celle, G. Aspetti anatomofunzionali della mucosa fundica in soggetti con carcinoma gastrico. *Rass. Ital. Gastroenterol.* 5 (1961):176–180.
26. De Boer, W. G. R. M., Forsyth, A., and Nairn, R. C. Gastric antigens in health and disease. Behaviour in early development, senescence, metaplasia and cancer. *Br. Med. J.* 3 (1969):93–94.
27. Stemmermann, G. N. Comparative study of histochemical patterns in non-neoplastic and neoplastic gastric epithelium. A study of Japanese in Hawaii. *J. Natl. Cancer Inst.* 39 (1967):375–382.
28. Tarpila, S., Telkkä, A., and Siurala, M. Ultrastructure of various metaplasias of the stomach. *Acta Pathol. Microbiol. Scand.* 77 (1969):187–195.
29. Croft, D. N., Pollock, D. J., and Coghill, N. F. Cell loss from human gastric mucosa measured by the estimation of deoxyribonucleic acid (DNA) in gastric washings. *Gut* 7 (1966):333–338.
30. Nagayo, T. Dysplastic changes of the digestive tract related to cancer. *Acta Endosc.* 10 (1980):69–79.
31. Cheli, R., and Giacosa A. Dysplasia and chronic gastritis of the fundic and antral mucosa. Abstracts of World Congress of Gastroenterology, Stockholm, 1982.

11 SIGNIFICANCE OF CHRONIC GASTRITIS AS A PRECANCEROUS CONDITION OF THE STOMACH

T. Hirota, R. Sano, M. Daibo, M. Itabashi, and H. Kitaoka

Although there have been many histological classifications of chronic gastritis offered by different investigators, Schindler's classification (1) has been used internationally. Sano (2) introduced a new classification based on his understanding of chronic gastritis as a reorganization phenomenon of the mucosal structure by regenerative activity after a defect of the gastric mucosal epithelium. His classification provided a quantitative subtyping of metaplastic gastritis.

Many researchers have reported a relation between gastric cancer and chronic gastritis, especially metaplastic gastritis. However, there are few reports that present the extent of chronic gastritis in the stomach and its association with gastric carcinoma. In the present chapter, we report the association of various gastric diseases, especially early gastric cancer, with each type of chronic gastritis according to Sano's classification (2) with a slight modification.

MATERIALS AND METHODS

The materials used for this study consisted of 1,439 surgically resected gastric specimens from the National Cancer Center in Tokyo, Japan, obtained during a period of 12 years from May 1962 to May 1974. The average age and the sex ratio of the patients with various diseases are shown in Table 11-1. The average age of patients with duodenal ulcers was 39 years, but those in the other groups were in their sixth or seventh decades. Regarding the sex of the patients, males comprised the majority of benign cases. Early gastric carcinoma had a higher frequency in males, twice that in females.

We have devised a rather unique and appropriate histologic technique. The resected stomach was cut into long, 0.5-centimeter-wide strips parallel to the lesser curvature. Paraffin sections were prepared as usual. The localization of benign or malignant lesions and the distribution of each type of chronic gastritis after Sano's classification (2) with a minor modification were schematically drawn after histological examination. This reconstructive method has the advantage of expressing the pattern of the distribution of chronic gastritis qualitatively and quantitatively.

The classification of chronic gastritis used in this study was as follows [Sano's classification (2) with a minor modification]. In metaplastic gastritis the gastric mucosa shows partial or complete intestinal metaplasia. There are three subtypes of metaplastic gastritis. In the wide type intestinal metaplasia is distributed in almost the whole stomach, involving the antrum and more than the lower half of the gastric body. The distribution of intestinal metaplasia in the intermediate type is limited to the area from the antrum to the transitional zone between the pyloric and fundic gland areas. In the antral type the intestinal me-

Table 11-1. Average Age and Sex Ratio in Various Diseases

	Duodenal Ulcer	Gastric Polyp	Gastric Ulcer	Early Gastric Cancer		Total
				With Ulcer	Without Ulcer	
No. of cases	281	123	435	406	194	1,439
Average age (years)	39.0	55.7	51.6	51.7	61.6	50.9
Sex ratio (male/female)	9.8	1.1	4.6	1.9	1.8	2.9

taplasia is limited to the antrum. Non-metaplastic gastritis consists of two types: atrophic and verrucous. In the atrophic type, non-meta-plastic atrophic mucosa is seen either throughout or only in parts of the stomach. Either hyperplasia of the pyloric glands in the antral area or hyperplasia of the foveolar epithelium in the gastric body is seen in the verrucous type.

RESULTS

Frequency of Chronic Gastritis Subtypes According to Age of Patients

All cases of stomachs resected for duodenal ulcers, gastric ulcers, gastric polyps, and early gastric cancers were histologically reviewed to determine the type of chronic gastritis. The frequency of each type of chronic gastritis appearing in patients grouped according to age (decades) is summarized in Figure 11-1. The incidence of metaplastic gas-

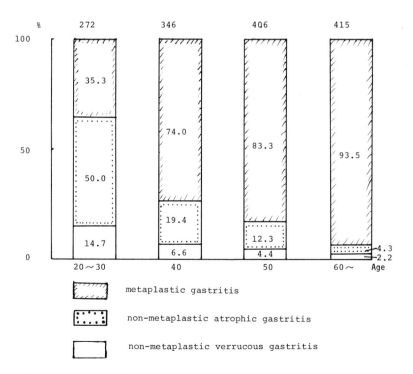

Figure 11-1. Frequency of subtypes of chronic gastritis according to age in resected stomachs with various diseases.

tritis was 35.3 percent in the third and fourth decades. It increased rapidly in the fifth decade up to 74.0 percent.

Frequency of Chronic Gastritis Subtypes

The incidence of metaplastic gastritis was 74.9 percent (See Table 11-2). Of the three subtypes, wide-type metaplastic gastritis was most common, appearing in 33.8 percent of cases; the intermediate type appeared in 26.8 percent and the antral type in 14.3 percent. Non-metaplastic atrophic gastritis was seen in 18.8 percent of cases and verrucous gastritis in only 6.3 percent.

Chronic Gastritis in Benign Cases

Chronic gastritis in gastric ulcer cases was mainly of the metaplastic type, seen in 84.1 percent of benign cases (Table 11-2). In the back-

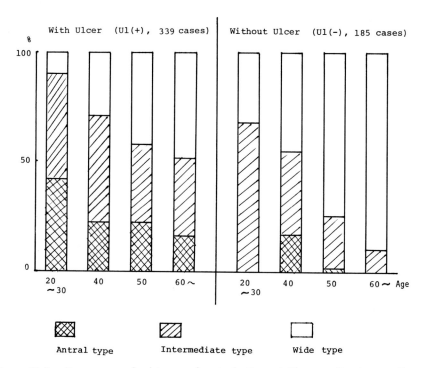

Figure 11-2. Frequency of subtypes of metaplastic gastritis according to age: Comparison between carcinoma with ulcer and carcinoma without ulcer.

Table 11-2. Distribution of Chronic Gastritis

Gastritis	Duodenal Ulcer (281)	Gastric Polyp (123)	Gastric Ulcer (435)	Early Gastric Cancer Ulcerated (406)	Early Gastric Cancer No Ulcer (194)	Total (1,439)
Metaplastic						
wide type	8.2	52.8	27.6	31.5	77.3	33.8
Intermediate						
type	20.6	8.9	33.8	34.5	15.5	26.8
Antral type	9.6	3.3	22.8	17.5	2.6	14.3
Nonmetaplastic						
Atrophic type	45.2	22.0	11.5	15.0	2.6	18.8
Verrucous type	16.4	13.0	4.3	1.5	2.0	6.3

Values are expressed as percentages of cases. Numbers in parentheses are numbers of cases.

ground gastric mucosa of benign gastric polyp and duodenal ulcer, non-metaplastic gastritis was seen in 35.0 and 61.6 percent of benign cases, respectively. Metaplastic gastritis was seen less frequently.

Chronic Gastritis in Cases with Early Gastric Cancer

The early gastric cancer cases were divided into two groups (Table 11-2). In one group of 406 cases, peptic ulcer or ulcer scar was present. In the other group of 194 cases, no ulcerative change was present. Metaplastic gastritis was associated frequently with early gastric cancer, especially with nonulcerative ones. Wide-type metaplastic gastritis was associated with carcinoma without ulcer twice as frequently as that with ulcer. The same tendency was also present even when compared between the same age groups (Figure 11-2). Nonmetaplastic atrophic gastritis was seen in 15.0 percent of cases with early gastric cancer with ulcer or ulcer scar and in 2.6 percent of those without ulcerative change.

DISCUSSION

There have been many reports (3–6) on the relation of gastric cancer to chronic gastritis, especially to metaplastic gastritis. Most of these studies were performed with biopsy or autopsy materials (7) and led to the conclusion that the incidence of intestinal metaplasia is parallel to that of gastric cancer. However, few reports presented a quantitative study of how widely chronic gastritis is distributed throughout the stomach. Therefore, in this study we used Sano's classification of chronic gastritis (2) with a slight modification in which a quantitative subclassification of metaplastic gastritis was provided. With this classification we examined the association of various benign and malignant gastric diseases with each type of chronic gastritis.

Early gastric carcinoma was divided into two types; one was associated with peptic ulcer or ulcer scar in the same lesion and the other with no ulcerative change. This was done in order to see if there was any difference between the two types and between benign and malignant ulcers in terms of association with types of gastritis. Our results revealed the most frequent association of carcinoma with metaplastic gastritis, especially with the wide type. It is noteworthy that carcinoma without ulcer was associated most frequently with the wide type of metaplastic gastritis. Carcinoma with ulcerative change showed less frequent association with the wide-type metaplastic gastritis than did nonulcerative carcinoma, but it was as frequent as benign gastric ulcer. Non-metaplastic gastritis as a background of early gastric carcinoma was found less frequently (21.1 percent of cases). However, when dividing carcinoma into the two subtypes, carcinoma with ulcer or ulcer scar was relatively more frequently (15 percent) associated with non-metaplastic gastritis than carcinoma without ulcer (2.6 percent). This suggests that there are different types of carcinoma in histological and biological character and that each of them may have different background conditions concerning chronic gastritis. Although metaplastic gastritis seems to be closely related to the occurrence of carcinoma, non-metaplastic gastritis can also be a precancerous condition. It is noteworthy that carcinoma occurs in the severely atrophic (non-metaplastic) gastric mucosa of patients with pernicious anemia more frequently than in the healthy population.

In benign gastric ulcer and gastric polyp cases, metaplastic gastritis also occurred most frequently, especially the wide and intermediate types. However, non-metaplastic gastritis was relatively more frequent in these benign lesions than carcinoma (in spite of the above evidence). In contrast to the gastric diseases mentioned above, non-metaplastic gastritis was remarkably frequent in duodenal ulcer cases. This may be due to the younger age of these patients compared with that of patients with gastric diseases.

From the frequent association of metaplastic gastritis with benign gastric ulcer and polyp, we cannot rule out the possibility that metaplastic gastritis simply accidentally accompanies the carcinoma. However, the higher frequency of association between carcinoma, especially the nonulcerative type, and the wide type of metaplastic gastritis strongly suggests a close relation between the two diseases. Further studies are necessary to determine whether metaplastic gastritis is a precancerous or paracancerous (induced by the same stimulants or under the same conditions that also induce carcinoma) condition or both. A detailed study of the spatial relation of carcinoma to subtypes (complete and incomplete) of metaplastic gastritis is described in Chapter 15.

SUMMARY

In order to clarify the significance of chronic gastritis as a precancerous condition of the stomach, 1,439 stomachs surgically resected for early gastric carcinoma (600 cases), benign gastric ulcer (435 cases), benign gastric polyps (123 cases), and duodenal ulcer (281 cases) were histologically examined. Sano's classification of chronic gastritis (2) with a minute modification was used. It consisted of metaplastic and non-metaplastic gastritis and the quantitative subclassification of metaplastic gastritis. Metaplastic gastritis was most frequent, corresponding to 74.9 percent of the total cases.

Carcinoma, benign gastric ulcer, benign gastric polyps, and duodenal ulcer were found to be associated with metaplastic gastritis in this decreasing order of frequency: 87.3, 84.1, 65.0, and 38.4 percent, respectively. Association of non-metaplastic gastritis with carcinoma was less frequent (12.7 percent). Metaplastic gastritis was associated more frequently with carcinoma without an ulcerative change in the same lesion (95.4 percent) than with carcinoma with ulcer (83.5 percent). The widely distributed type of metaplastic gastritis showed a higher association with carcinoma than the other subtypes. The results of the present study suggest that there is a certain close relation between gastric carcinoma and metaplastic gastritis, especially between carcinoma without ulcerative change and the wide type of metaplastic gastritis. Further study is needed to determine whether metaplastic gastritis is a precancerous or paracancerous condition.

ACKNOWLEDGMENTS

The authors are indebted to Dr. Si-Chun Ming, Professor at Temple University, Philadelphia, Pennsylvania, for his helpful suggestions and revising the manuscript. We are much obliged to Drs. H. Kobayashi, K. Maekawa, M. Ono, Y. Izumi, T. Shimoda, and Y. Yamamoto for their contribution in the histological examinations. We thank Mrs. S. Matsuoka and Miss Y. Yamauchi for their skillful technical assistance. We are also obliged to the members of the gastrointestinal tract study group of the National Cancer Center Hospital, Tokyo.

This work was supported in part by Grants-in-Aid for Cancer Research from the Ministry of Education (grant no. 58010091).

REFERENCES

1. Schindler, R. Die chronische gastritis. *Klin. Wochenschr.* 44 (1966):601.
2. Sano, R. *Surgical Pathology of Gastric Diseases*, pp. 139–205. Tokyo: Igaku Shoin Ltd., 1974.
3. Correa, P., Cuello, C., and Duque, E. Carcinoma and intestinal metaplasia of the stomach of Colombian migrants. *J. Natl. Cancer Inst.* 44 (1970):297–306.
4. Imai, T., Kubo, T., and Watanabe, T. Chronic gastritis in Japanese with reference to high incidence of gastric carcinoma. *J. Natl. Cancer Inst.* 47 (1971):179–195.
5. Kubo, T., and Imai, T. A geographic-pathological study of intestinal metaplasia of the gastric mucosa—Comparison with autopsy cases between Chilean and New Zealand people. *Trans. Soc. Pathol. Jpn.* 64 (1975):208.
6. Tanigawa, H., Yamazaki, S., Morita, M., Yamazaki, Y., and Konishi, T. A case report of pernicious anemia associated with multiple early gastric cancer. *Stomach Intest.* 12 (1977):785–791.
7. Bonne, C., Hartz, H., Klerks, J. V., Posthuma, J. H., and Radsma, W. Morphology of the stomach and gastric secretion in Malays and Chinese and the different incidence of gastric ulcer and cancer in these races. *Am. J. Cancer* 33 (1938):265–280.

IV INTESTINAL METAPLASIA

12 INTESTINAL METAPLASIA: ITS HETEROGENEOUS NATURE AND SIGNIFICANCE

S.-C Ming

Intestinal metaplasia occurs frequently in the stomach, particularly in certain diseases. The most common associated condition is chronic atrophic gastritis. For instance, in the group of patients with chronic atrophic gastritis followed by Siurala (1), 89 percent developed intestinal metaplasia in about 20 years. Such a study also illustrates that intestinal metaplasia is an acquired disease rather than a congenital heterotopia. Intestinal metaplasia has also been postulated to be a causative factor for gastric ulcer and carcinoma. The latter possibility was proposed by Morson (2) in 1955. The evidences for it are found in the high frequency of intestinal metaplasia in cancerous stomachs and the development of carcinoma in the metaplastic epithelium. This concept was enhanced by the proposal of Lauren (3) in 1965 to divide gastric carcinomas into two major types: intestinal and diffuse. The cancer cells in the intestinal type of carcinoma have many features of intestinal cells, and the histological pattern of the carcinoma resembles that of colonic carcinoma. At the same time, however, Lauren (3) pointed out that many carcinomas of the diffuse type also have characteristics of intestinal cells. This observation has been confirmed by various studies including electron microscopy and histochemistry. (4, 5). The current view is that while both the intestinal and diffuse types of gastric carcinoma have intestinal features, the intestinal type of cancer, which is well differentiated, is much more closely related to intestinal metaplasia than the diffuse type. The evidences for this conclusion are the common occurrence of intestinal metaplasia in the vicinity of cancer, including early cancers (3, 6–8), and the high rate of dysplasia in intestinal metaplasia when it is associated with the intestinal type of cancer (9).

Various investigations including ultrastructural and histochemical ones have found that the metaplastic epithelium usually resembles the epithelium of the small intestine. However, in 1967, Ming et al. (10) noticed that in some instances the metaplastic process might be incomplete, in that instead of absorptive cells, the columnar cells between goblet cells had mucus secretion. The mucus granules were located in the apical portion of the cell, as in normal foveolar cells. However, the morphology of the granules indicated the presence of both gastric and intestinal mucus. Thus, in the incompletely metaplastic epithelium, the intervening columnar cells superficially resemble the foveolar cells, but in reality they are also metaplastic in terms of the nature of mucus secretion. In recent years the concept of incomplete metaplasia has been further extended and seriously implicated in carcinogenesis of the stomach (11–14).

It is now clear that intestinal metaplasia is a complicated process, and that the metaplastic cells are heterogeneous. It has therefore been divided into various types. The roles of the different types of intestinal metaplasia in gastric carcinogenesis are discussed in other chapters. In this chapter the basis of classification and the relation between gastric carcinoma and intestinal metaplasia are reviewed.

METHODS OF INVESTIGATION

Careful microscopic examination of a routinely prepared tissue section is adequate to identify a metaplastic epithelium. Instead of a continuous mucous cell layer lining the surface and foveolae of a normal stomach, the metaplastic epithelium is characterized by the presence of goblet cells and intervening columnar cells, which may be mucus secreting or non–mucus secreting (Figures 12-1 and Plate 12-1). The non-mucus secreting cells may or may not have a distinct striated border. Paneth cells are also easily recognized. Other techniques are

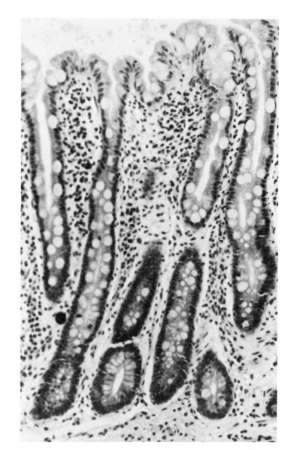

Figure 12-1. Complete metaplasia in chronic atrophic gastritis. The metaplastic epithelium is composed of goblet cells and non-mucus-secreting absorptive cells. Mitoses are present in the lower portion of the glands. H&E stain. × 200.

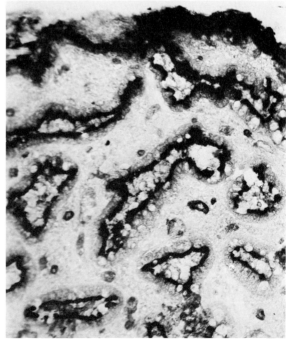

Figure 12-2. Alkaline phosphatase (black) along the luminal surface of completely metaplasic cells. It is also present in the endothelium. × 200.

needed to bring out detailed cellular characteristics. The most commonly used method is mucin histochemistry. More recently, immunological techniques have also been applied.

Mucin Histochemistry

The mucus secreted by the epithelial cells of the gastrointestinal tract falls into three major categories: neutral glycoprotein, sialomucin, and sulfomucin. Sialomucin may be subdivided into N-acylated and O-acylated types. The commonly used histochemical stains used to identify them are: periodic acid-Schiff reaction (PAS)—stains all mucus red (15; Plate 12-2); alcian blue (AB)—stains sulfomucins (at pH 1.0) and sialomucins (at pH 2.5) blue (15); periodate borohydride/potassium hydroxide/PAS (Pb/KOH/PAS)—stains O-acylated sialomucins red (16); and high-iron diamine/AB (HID/AB)—stains sulfomucin brown-black and sialomucin blue (17).

A combination of these techniques may be used on a single specimen to demonstrate various mucins (18). Examples of staining results are shown in Plates 12-2 to 12-8.

The distribution of the various types of mucosubstances in the normal gastrointestinal tract is listed in Table 12-1.

Enzyme Histochemistry

The microvilli of the absorptive cells of the small intestine have a number of enzymes such as peptidases, disaccharidases, and alkaline phosphatases. These enzymes are absent in the normal stomach and are sporadically present in the normal colon. These enzymes have therefore been used to identify intestinal metaplasia (18, 19). Alkaline phosphatase (Figure 12-2) and aminopeptidase have been found to be most useful (19). Cytoplasmic enzymes such as dehydrogenases and hydrolases are nonspecific but often stronger in the metaplastic cells than in gastric cells (18).

Enzymes can also be demonstrated in gross specimens. For instance, alkaline phosphatase has been shown by Stemmermann and

Table 12-1. Distribution of Mucin in Normal Gastrointestinal Tract

Mucin	Location
Neutral glycoprotein	Stomach
Sialomucin, N-acylated	Some deep foveolae; all small intestine; proximal colon
Sialomucin, O-acylated	Some foveolae; duodenum and distal ileum; colon
Sulfomucin	Some deep foveolae; colon; terminal ileum

Table 12-2. Enzyme Histochemistry

	AP		LAP		EST		SDH		DD	
	+	+ +	+	+ +	+	+ +	+	+ +	+	+ +
Stomach										
Normal (55)	0	0	0	0	38	49	16	73	55	45
Metaplasia										
Complete (10)	30	70	50	50	0	100	0	100	0	100
Incomplete (5)	40	0	80	0	100	0	100	0	100	0
Carcinoma (14)	0	21	14	43	7	93	36	64	0	100
Small intestine (24)	0	100	0	100	0	100	0	100	0	100
Colon (46)	46	15	20	13	17	83	0	100	4	96

AP, alkaline phosphatase; LAP, leucine aminopeptidase; EST, nonspecific esterase; SDH, succinic dehydrogenase; DD, DPNH diaphorase; +, weakly positive; + +, strongly positive.

Numbers in parentheses are the numbers of specimens. All values are expressed as percentages.

Source: This work was done in collaboration with Harvey Goldman at Beth Israel Hospital, Boston, Massachusetts.

Hayashi (20) to be related to gastric cancer as well as ulcer. Others have used the Tes-Tape method to demonstrate alkaline phosphatase, aminopeptidase, and disaccharidases (13, 21). The distribution of some enzymes is shown in Table 12-2.

Electron Microscopy

Ultrastructural features of well-developed metaplastic cells resemble those of the epithelial cells of the small intestine (10, 22). The incompletely metaplastic epithelium is lined by goblet and mucous columnar cells. The latter have mixed types of mucin granules and poorly developed microvilli (10). Furthermore, Paneth cells are absent, and endocrine and goblet cells are fewer (23).

Immunohistochemistry

Immunohistochemical studies have recently been used to detect mucin-related antigens in gastric tissue, both benign and malignant. A goblet cell antigen purified from a signet-ring cell carcinoma of the stomach has been found in the goblet cells of normal intestine, metaplastic stomach, and colonic as well as gastric carcinomas, indicating a link among them (24). An antigen specific for colon and fetal duodenum (M3C) is present in some gastric cancers and in the metaplastic epithelium adjacent to cancer, whereas the metaplastic epithelium of benign stomachs has only antigens of small intestine (M3SI) and adult duodenum (M3D), indicating a relationship between the fetal status of metaplastic epithelium and cancer (25).

CLASSIFICATION OF INTESTINAL METAPLASIA

Based primarily on light microscopy and histochemical studies, intestinal metaplasia has been classified into complete and incomplete types (11, 13, 14). Based on mucin histochemistry alone, it has been classified into small intestinal and colonic types, or a type secreting sulfomucin and a type not secreting sulfomucin (12, 26–28). The criteria for classification are not always the same. For instance, incomplete metaplasia has been defined as one without Paneth cells (29), lacking certain enzymes (13), and with the presence of mucous cells in place of absorptive cells (13, 14). The types of mucin used for separating small intestinal and colonic types of metaplasia were also different (26–28). There is a need for a unified concept for classification.

It is clear that metaplasia is an abnormal process. Therefore, it is a form of dysplasia in the broad sense. The metaplastic epithelium is different from the normal gastrointestinal epithelium. For instance, the metaplastic epithelium does not form well-defined villi and crypts as in the normal small intestine, nor does it contain the same number of goblet and absorptive cells as the normal colon. The presence of mucous columnar cells is definitely abnormal. Therefore, the classification of metaplasia has to be based on certain key factors rather than on the entire composition of the epithelium. In this regard, the type of mucin seems to be a reliable marker, since its distribution pattern in the normal gastrointestinal tract appears constant. The concept of complete and incomplete types of metaplasia also needs updating. The latter (10) was based on the supposition that the cells between the goblet cells were normal foveolar cells and that the gland was only partially replaced by the intestinal type of cells. Recent studies have shown that the mucous columnar cells (as distinct from goblet and foveolar cells) may contain a large amount of acidic mucin not present in the normal foveolar cells, although they look like foveolar cells. Under electron microscopy they are seen to have more and better-developed microvilli (22). Thus, these cells are in fact metaplastic cells with mixed features of foveolar, absorptive, and goblet cells. As to be expected, the enzyme pattern of both types of metaplasia falls in between that of stomach and intestine (Table 12-2).

Another set of criteria is morphological. The epithelium of normal small intestine is characterized by the presence of absorptive and

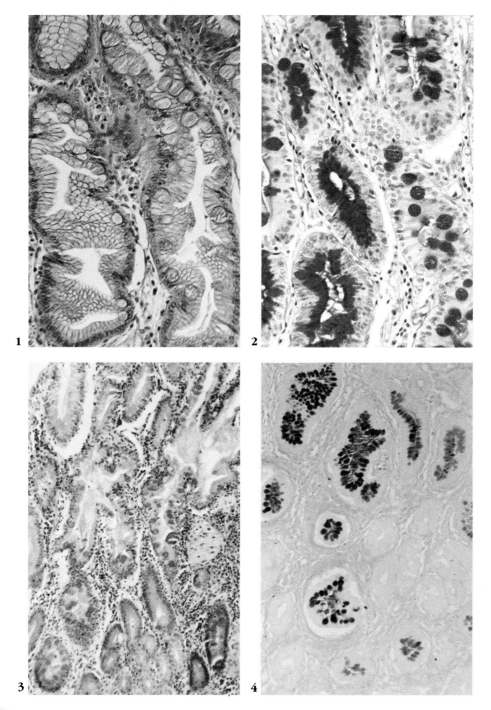

Plate 12-1. Incomplete metaplasia. The mucus globules in the goblet cells are slightly basophilic, indicating an acidic nature. The intervening columnar cells resemble normal foveolar mucous cells and do not have striated borders. H&E stain. × 360. **Plate 12-2.** The glands on the right are completely metaplastic, showing red-staining mucus in the goblet cells and distinct striated borders, also stained red, on absorptive cells. The glands on the left are incompletely metaplastic, showing goblet cells and mucous columnar cells with varying amounts of mucus. PAS stain. × 360. **Plate 12-3.** Complete and incomplete metaplasia. The mucus globules in the goblet cells are stained deep red. The mucus in some foveolar cells is stained light pink. PB/KOH/PAS stain. × 125. **Plate 12-4.** Complete metaplasia. The mucus in the goblet cells is stained brown-black (sulfomucin), blue (sialomucin), or a combination of both. Gastric glands are unstained. HID/AB stain. × 90.

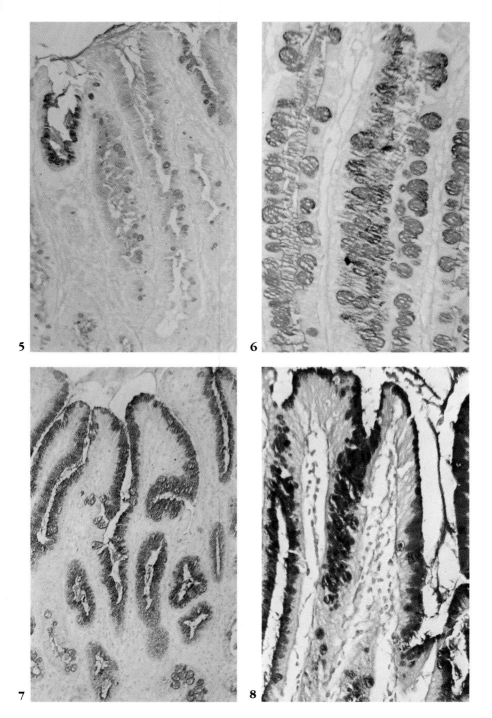

Plate 12-5. Incomplete metaplasia. The mucin in the goblet cells is stained deep blue (sialomucin). The mucous columnar cells are stained light blue (small intestinal type of incomplete metaplasia). The mucous columnar cells of the gland at the upper left corner are stained brown-black (colonic type of incomplete metaplasia). HID/AB stain. × 180. **Plate 12-6.** Complete and incomplete metaplasia in the same glands. The goblet cells contain mainly sialomucin (blue). The mucous columnar cells contain mostly sulfomucin (brown). Thus the colonic type of incomplete metaplasia coexists with the small intestinal type of complete metaplasia. HID/AB stain. × 360. **Plate 12-7.** AB(pH 2.5)/PAS combination stain showing coexistence of different types of metaplasia. The red-stained glycoprotein is present only in the foveolar cells (*upper right*) and some mucous columnar cells (*midright*). Most mucous columnar cells in incompletely metaplastic glands have a mixture of neutral and acid mucins. The goblet cells in both complete and incomplete metaplastic glands have blue-stained sialomucin. × 90. **Plate 12-8.** HID/AB/PAS combination stain showing both gastric and colonic types of incomplete metaplasia with red glycoprotein or brown sulfomucin in the mucous columnar cells. The goblet cells contain both sialo- and sulfomucin with blue-brown granules. × 180.

Table 12-3. Types and Main Features of Intestinal Metaplasia

| | Complete Type | | Incomplete Type | | |
	Small Intestinal	Colonic	Gastric	Small Intestinal	Colonic
Cells					
Absorptive cells	+	+	0	0	0
Striated border	+	0	0	0	0
Mucous columnar cells	0	0	+	+	+
Goblet cells	+	+	+	+	+
Paneth cells	+	0	0	0	0
Mucins in goblet cells					
Neutral glycoprotein	0	0	0	0	0
Sialomucin, *N*-acylated	+	0	+	+	+
Sialomucin, *O*-acylated	V	+	0	V	V
Sulfomucin	0	+	V	+	+
Mucins in mucous columnar cells					
Neutral glycoprotein	N	N	+	V	V
Sialomucin, *N*-acylated	N	N	0	+	V
Sialomucin, *O*-acylated	N	N	0	0	V
Sulfomucin	N	N	0	0	+

+ , present; 0, mostly absent; V, variable; N, not applicable.

goblet cells lining the villus and immature, mucous, Paneth, and endo-crine cells in the crypt. In the metaplastic epithelium, Paneth cells may be absent and the number of endocrine cells low. This situation is found in the incompletely metaplastic epithelium, but may also be found in an epithelium without mucous columnar cells. The latter situation is present in the normal colon.

When all the above factors are taken into consideration, the metaplastic epithelium can be classified into five types, as shown in Table 12-3, depending on the dominant features. The major categories of complete and incomplete types are distinguished by the absence and presence, respectively, of mucous columnar cells. The complete type is separated into small intestinal and colonic subtypes. The colonic type has sulfomucin, an ill-defined striated border, and no Paneth cells. The small intestinal type has sialomucin, a distinct striated border, and Paneth cells. The subtypes of incomplete epithelium are determined by the type of mucin in the mucous columnar cells, since the staining characteristics of their goblet cells are similar. These types often coexist in the same stomach. Examples are shown in Plates 12-2 to 12-8.

SIGNIFICANCE OF INTESTINAL METAPLASIA AS A PRECANCEROUS LESION

Gastric cancer cells often have the subcellular features possessed by intestinal cells, such as microvilli, acidic mucin, and digestive enzymes. These features suggest the possibility that gastric carcinomas originate from intestinalized cells rather than gastric cells. This possibility is supported by the frequent association of intestinal metaplasia with carcinoma (Figure 12-3). On the other hand, intestinal metaplasia is a very common phenomenon. The malignant potential of the metaplastic epithelium must be small. The question of the relationship between intestinal metaplasia and cancer lay dormant until recently when the incomplete type of metaplasia was brought to the forefront.

In 1976 Kawachi et al. (30) divided intestinal metaplasia into complete and incomplete types and found them to be related to gastric cancer in 55 and 41 cases, respectively. Since then various reports have implicated the incomplete type more heavily than the complete type in gastric carcinogenesis (11, 13, 14, 29) and the colonic or sulfomucin-producing type over other types (12, 26–28). Most of these reports also emphasize that the intestinal and well-differentiated glandular carcinoma is more closely related to metaplasia than the diffuse and poorly differentiated carcinoma. It should be noted, however, that the differences are only in term of relativeness.

Close and frequent association does not indicate a causal relationship, even when the association is noted in cases of very small early cancer. In fact, study of such cases has shown that carcinoma may have several starting points, and that the metaplastic epithelium is only one of them (31).

Gastric carcinoma can be easily produced in animals by feeding N-methyl-N'-nitro-N-nitrosoguanidine in the drinking water. Intestinal metaplasia occurs infrequently in such experiments (32, 33). A recent experimental study further identifies the induced carcinoma as of gastric cell origin, although intestinal metaplasia is also present (34).

In view of these findings, it may be concluded that intestinal metaplasia, particularly the incomplete and colonic types, is a cancer-associated condition but not necessarily a precancerous lesion. In order to be precancerous, the metaplastic epithelium has to become dysplastic (see Chapter 2). It is likely that metaplasia is one of the effects of carcinogenic stimulation, and malignant as well as benign cells may pursue various lines of metaplastic change under such an influence.

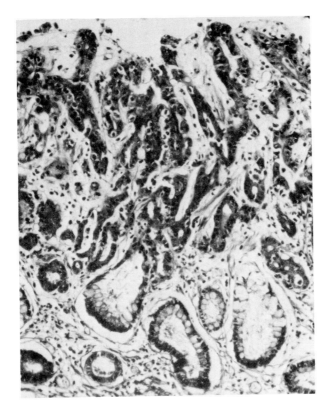

Figure 12-3. An early gastric carcinoma of the intestinal type in a metaplastic epithelium. × 150.

DISCUSSION

One question raised in the past was why carcinoma developed more frequently in the metaplastic gastric mucosa than in the normal small intestine. The question is no longer valid because the metaplastic mucosa is an abnormal mucosa and not merely a misplaced small intestine mucosa in the stomach. Furthermore, it has not been proven that carcinoma develops more frequently from the metaplastic than from the gastric cell—certainly not in experimental animals where a sequential study of the carcinogenic process is possible. The experimental model, in fact, indicates only a coincidental rather than a causal relationship between metaplasia and cancer (34). The same relationship may exist in humans as suggested before (10).

Intestinal metaplasia is commonly seen in various gastric conditions. It can probably be caused by multiple different agents. Carcinogenic stimulation may be one of them. Under such stimulation, the injured gastric epithelium regenerates into an abnormal, i.e., meta-

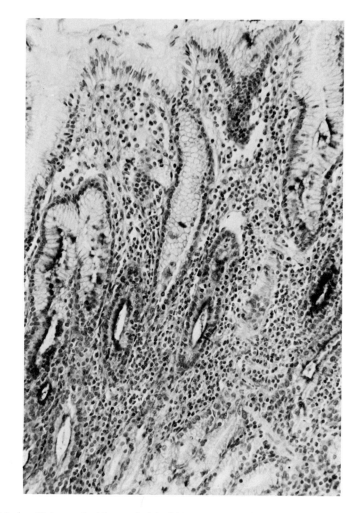

Figure 12-4.   Sialomucin (shown in black) is present in the deep foveolar cells of this stomach with chronic gastritis. The positive cells are immature low columnar cells, some of which are in mitosis. AB(pH 2.5) stain. × 215.

plastic, or a cancerous tissue. The metaplastic tissue already affected by the carcinogen may develop cancer at a faster or more frequent rate. Such sequences may be, but have not been, evaluated under experimental conditions.

There appears to be a close relationship between the secretion of sulfomucin and cancer. Previous studies have shown that the deep foveolar cells in the antrum often secrete sulfomucin (15), usually in the presence of severe gastritis (Figure 12–4). Sulfomucin secretion by foveolar cells may be indicative of an immature state, occurring at the time of cell regeneration following injury. The same may be true for the metaplastic epithelium. The mucosa adjacent to a cancer is usually severely inflamed and therefore more likely to secrete sulfomucin. Sulfomucin may also be a marker for the fetal status of the epithelium, comparable to M3C antigen, which is present in the colon and fetal duodenum (25). Such an epithelium may be more susceptible to carcinogenic influence. In either case sulfomucin can be viewed as a marker for a mucosa that may be the seat of a cancer.

Incomplete metaplasia is unique. It has rarely been reported in experimental studies, probably because it has escaped attention. What is postulated for sulfomucin may apply here also: namely, the sulfomucin-secreting mucous columnar cells are indeed immature foveolar cells in a regenerating state. If that is the case, the incompletely metaplastic epithelium is in fact a partially metaplastic epithelium. Its high frequency of association with carcinoma may be explained in the same way as sulfomucin.

Up to now, intestinal metaplasia has been extensively studied only in resected specimens. The high association rate between metaplasia and cancer may be due simply to a parallel or coincidental induction of both by the same carcinogenic stimulus. In this case metaplasia is a marker of carcinogenesis.

Metaplasia is certainly not a prerequisite precancerous lesion. Cancer develops often in the nonmetaplastic gastric mucosa in both humans and animals. The question of whether cancer develops more readily in a metaplastic mucosa, whatever its cause or causes, has not been dealt with adequately. Prospective study using gastroscopic biopsy will be a very valuable instrument to evaluate this problem. Such a study will not only elucidate the role of different types of metaplasia in gastric carcinogenesis, but will also determine the frequency and the latent duration of cancer development.

REFERENCES

1. Siurala, M. Gastritis, its fate and sequelae. *Ann. Clin. Res.* 13 (1981):111–113.
2. Morson, B. C. Carcinoma arising from areas of intestinal metaplasia in the gastric mucosa. *Br. J. Cancer* 9 (1955):377–385.
3. Lauren, P. The two histological main types of gastric carcinoma: Diffuse and so-called intestinal type carcinoma. An attempt at a histoclinical classification. *Acta Pathol. Microbiol. Scand.* 64 (1965):31–49.
4. Nevaläinen, T. J., and Järvi, O. H. Ultrastructure of intestinal and diffuse type gastric carcinoma. *J. Pathol.* 122 (1977):129–136.
5. Kobori, O., and Oota, K. Mucous substance and enzyme histochemistry of non-neoplastic and neoplastic gastric epithelium in man. *Acta Pathol. Jpn.* 24 (1974):119–130.
6. Stemmermann, G., Haenszel, W., and Locke, F. Epidemiologic pathology of gastric ulcer and gastric carcinoma among Japanese in Hawaii. *J. Natl. Cancer Inst.* 58 (1977):13–20.

7. Oohara, T., Tohma, H., Takezoe, K., Ukawa, S., Johjima, Y., Asakura, R., Aono, G., and Kurosaka, H. Minute gastric cancers less than 5 mm in diameter. *Cancer* 50 (1982):801–810.

8. Hirota, T., Itabashi, M., Suzuki, K., and Yoshida, S. Clinicopathologic study of minute and small early gastric cancer. Histogenesis of gastric cancer. *Pathol. Annu.* 15 (1980):1–19.

9. Ming, S.-C. Dysplasia of gastric epithelium. *Front. Gastrointest. Res.* 4 (1979):164–172.

10. Ming, S. -C., Goldman, H., and Frieman, D. G. Intestinal metaplasia and histogenesis of carcinoma in human stomach. Light and electron microscopic study. *Cancer* 20 (1967):1418–1429.

11. Jass, J. R. Role of intestinal metaplasia in the histogenesis of gastric carcinoma. *J. Clin. Pathol.* 33 (1980):801–810.

12. Jass, J. R., and Filipe, M. I. The mucin profiles of normal gastric mucosa, intestinal metaplasia and its variants and gastric carcinoma. *Histochem. J.* 13 (1981): 931–939.

13. Matsukura, N., Suzuki, K., Kawachi, T., Aoyagi, M., Sugima, T., Kifaoka, H., Numajiri, H., Shirota, A., Itabashi, M., and Hirota, T. Distribution of marker enzymes and mucin in intestinal metaplasia in human stomach and relation of complete and incomplete types of intestinal metaplasia to minute gastric carcinomas. *J. Natl. Cancer Inst.* 65 (1980):231–240.

14. Iida, F., and Kusama, J. Gastric carcinoma and intestinal metaplasia: Significance of types of intestinal metaplasia upon development of gastric carcinoma. *Cancer* 50 (1982):2854–2858.

15. Goldman, H., and Ming, S. -C. Mucins in normal and neoplastic gastrointestinal epithelium. Histochemical distribution. *Arch. Pathol.* 85 (1968):580–586.

16. Culling, C. F. A., Reid, P. E., Burton, J. D., and Dunn, W. L. A histochemical method of differentiating lower gastrointestinal tract mucin from other mucins in primary or metastatic tumors. *J. Clin. Pathol.* 28 (1975):656–658.

17. Spicer, S. S. Diamine methods for differentiating mucosubstances histochemically. *J. Histochem. Cytochem.* 13 (1965):211–234.

18. Abe, M., Ohuchi, N., and Sakano, H. Enzyme histo- and biochemistry of intestinalized gastric mucosa. *Acta Histochem. Cytochem.* 7 (1974):282–288.

19. Klein, N. C., Sleisenger, M. H., and Weser, E. Disaccharidases, leucine aminopeptidase and glucose uptake in intestinalized gastric mucosa and in gastric carcinoma. *Gastroenterology* 55 (1968):61–67.

20. Stemmermann, G. N., and Hayashi, T. Intestinal metaplasia of the gastric mucosa: A gross and microscopic study of its distribution in various disease states. *J. Natl. Cancer Inst.* 41 (1968):627–634.

21. Nomura, H. Histoenzymologic study of intestinal metaplasia of the gastric mucosa of resected gastric cancer tissue. II. Histologic findings. *Nippon Geka Gakkai Zasshi.* 80 (1979):500–511.

22. Goldman, H., and Ming, S. -C. Fine structure of intestinal metaplasia and adenocarcinoma of the human stomach. *Lab. Invest.* 18 (1968):203–210.

23. Intabashi, M., Hirota, T., Ohnuki, T., Matsuoka, S., Matsukura, N., Kawchi, T., Sugimura, T., and Kitaoka, H. Electron microscopic study of complete and incomplete types of intestinal metaplasia of the human gastric mucosa. *Proc. Jpn. Cancer Assoc.* p. 256, 1979.

24. Rapp, W., and Wurster, K. Alcian blue staining intestinal goblet cell antigen (GOA): A marker for gastric signet ring cell and colonic colloidal carcinoma. *Klin. Wochenschr.* 56 (1978):1185–1187.

25. Nardelli, J., Bara, J., Rosa, B., and Burtin, P. Intestinal metaplasia and carcinomas of the human stomach: An immunohistological study. *J. Histochem. Cytochem.* 31 (1983):366–375.

26. Teglbjaerg, P. S., and Nielsen, H. O. "Small intestinal type" and "colonic type" intestinal metaplasia of the human stomach, and their relationship to the histogenetic types of gastric adenocarcinoma. *Acta Pathol. Microbiol. Scand. (A)* 86 (1978):351–355.

27. Pagnini, C. A., and Bozzola, L. Precancerous significance of colonic type intestinal metaplasia. *Tumori* 69 (1981):113–116.

28. Sipponen, P., Seppälä, K., Varis, K., Hjelt, L., Ihamäki, T., Kekki, M., and Siurala, M. Intestinal metaplasia with colonic-type sulphomucins in the gastric mucosa; its association with gastric carcinoma. *Acta Pathol. Microbiol. Scand. (A)* 88 (1980): 217–224.

29. Onuma, C., Hirota, T., Itabashi, M., Misaka, R., Yoshida, H., Unagami, M., Oguro, Y., Yoshimori, M., Kitaoka, H., Kawachi, T., and Matsukura, N. Spatial relation between gastric atypical epithelium and subtypes of intestinal metaplasia. *Prog. Dig. Endosc.* 17 (1980):115–124.

30. Kawachi, T., Kurisu, M., Numanyu, N., Sasajima, K., and Sano, T. Precancerous changes in the stomach. *Cancer Res.* 36 (1976):2673–2677.

31. Schlake, W., and Grundmann, E. Multifocal early gastric cancer of mixed type. *Pathol. Res. Pract.* 164 (1979):331–341.

32. Saito, T., Sasaki, O., Tamada, R., Iwamatsu, M., and Inokuchi, K. Sequential studies of development of gastric carcinoma in dogs induced by N-methyl-N'-nitro-N-nitrosoguanidine. *Cancer* 42 (1978):1246–1254.

33. Sigaran, M. F., and Con-Wong, R. Production of proliferative lesions in gastric mucosa of albino mice by oral administration of N-methyl-N'-nitro-N-nitrosoguanidine. *Gann* 70 (1979):343–352.

34. Tatematsu, M., Furihata, C., Katsuyama, T., Hasegawa, R., Nakanowatari, J., Saito, D., Takahashi, M., Matsushima, T., and Ito, M. Independent induction of intestinal metaplasia and gastric cancer in rats treated with N-methyl-N'-nitro-N-nitrosoguanidine. *Cancer Res.* 43 (1983):1335–1341.

13 THE DYSPLASTIC NATURE OF INTESTINAL METAPLASIA IN THE STOMACH

G. N. Stemmermann, T. Hayashi, and S. Teruya

Intestinal metaplasia of the stomach may be defined as the replacement of antral or oxyntic gastric mucosa by glands composed of epithelium resembling that of the small intestine. This anatomic change is frequently encountered in populations at high risk for gastric cancer (1) and for gastric ulcer (2). It may be induced by chemical and physical agents that also cause gastric cancer, such as methylnitrosoguanidine (3) and X-irradiation (4). Nakamura et al. have observed that small intestinal-type cancers of the stomach are almost always associated with severe intestinal metaplasia (5). Intestinal metaplasia does not always precede or accompany gastric cancer in the experimental animal (6); and minute human gastric cancers may arise in the absence of intestinal metaplasia (7); and even when associated with metaplasia, a cancer may arise in an apparently nonmetaplastic area. These divergent experiences call into question whether intestinal metaplasia is a precursor to gastric cancer or a coincidental event unrelated to cancer induction. We have observed structural fea-

Table 13-1. Differences between Epithelium of Small Bowel and
That of Intestinal Metaplasia

Histologic Structure	Small Intestine Crypts and Villi	Intestinal Metaplasia Glands, No Villi
Microvilli		
enzymes	Uniformly found in all cells	Random cell-to-cell deletion
	Uniform distribution in duodenum and jejunum	Site-dependent deletion within stomach
"Bushy" microvilli	Absent	May be present
Cytoplasm		
mucus	Uniformly alcian blue positive	Site-dependent variation between alcian blue and high-iron diamine positive
Mucous Paneth cell hybrids	Absent	Present
Intracytoplasmic cysts with microvilli	Absent	Present
Cilia	Absent	May be present and dysplastic
Paneth cells		
distribution	All glands	Site-dependent deletion
location	Crypts	Basal or superior aspects if atypia present
DNA synthesis	Absent or infrequent	Common

tures of intestinal types of epithelium in the stomach that can best be termed "dysplastic." These features clearly distinguish the metaplastic epithelium from the mucosa of the small intestine, and probably represent a stage in the development of those antral cancers that are encountered in national populations at high risk for this tumor. The differences between metaplastic and small bowel mucosa are compared in Table 13-1 and are discussed in detail below.

STRUCTURAL FEATURES

Distribution

Intestinal metaplasia is, almost without exception, associated with gastritis. The distribution of the metaplastic process in the stomach depends upon the nature of this gastritis (Table 13-2). In national populations at high risk for gastric cancer, the process begins at the junc-

Table 13-2. Gastritis and Associated Factors

	Type A Gastritis	Type B Gastritis	Gastroenter-ostomy
Geographic association	Northern Europeans	Eastern Europe; Northeast Asia; Andean Highlands	— None
Gastric HCl	Decreased or absent	Decreased in late stages	Normal or decreased
Salt intake	No association	Increased	No association
NO$_3$ intake	No association	Increased	No association
Fruits and vegetables	No association	Decreased intake	No association
N-Nitroso compounds	In gastric juice	In mucosal homogenates and gastric juice	In gastric juice
Superficial gastritis	Constant in corpus; absent in antrum	Constant in antrum and corpus	Constant in gastric remnant
Intestinal metaplasia	Oxyntic mucosa	Antral and oxyntic mucosa	Inconstant

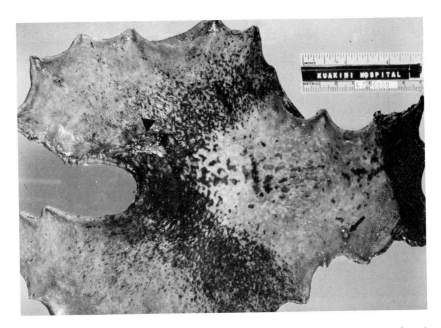

Figure 13-1.   Resected stomach stained for alkaline phosphatase activity, showing intestinal metaplasia at the junction of the antrum and corpus and along the lesser curvature. There is an ulcer (*triangle*) on the posterior wall in the metaplastic mucosa and a hyperplastic polyp (*arrow*) in the nonintestinalized antrum.

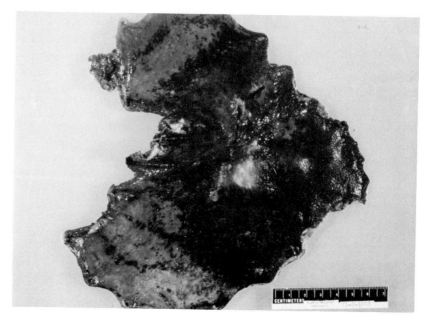

Figure 13-2.   Totally intestinalized antrum, showing extension of the process into the corpus. There is a carcinoma (*arrow*) on the posterior wall of the antrum. Stomach stained for alkaline phosphatase activity.

tion of the antrum and oxyntic mucosa. Later it may extend distally to involve the entire antrum and into the oxyntic mucosa that lines the whole of the proximal lesser curvature. In the last stages of this process, it may extend into the remainder of the oxyntic mucosa as fingerlike processes that follow the longitudinal mucosal folds. In contrast, the intestinal metaplasia associated with pernicious anemia is limited to the atrophic oxyntic mucosa. The glycocalyx of the metaplastic epithelium contains enzymes not normally found in the stomach. These enzymes have been used to make grossly visible maps of the distribution of intestinal metaplasia: alkaline phosphatase (8), various disaccharidases (9), and aminopeptidase (10). Some of the different patterns of alkaline phosphatase distribution in the stomach are shown in Figures 13-1 to 13-3.

Enzyme Histochemistry

The distribution of the glycocalyceal enzymes is uniform throughout the small intestine, but not in the metaplastic mucosa of the stomach.

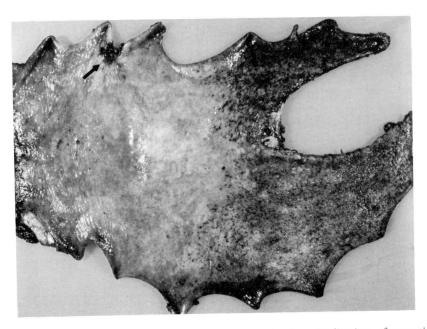

Figure 13-3. Stomach showing characteristic patchy intestinalization of oxyntic mucosa owing to pernicious anemia. There is a small carcinoma (*arrow*) on the greater curvature of the nonintestinalized antrum. Stomach stained for alkaline phosphatase activity. The positive stain of the center of the carcinoma is due to the presence of the enzyme in capillaries of the granulation tissue of the ulcerated central aspect of the tumor.

Kumagae (11) noted that alkaline phosphatase may be present in one metaplastic cell and absent from its immediate neighbor. We have confirmed this (Figure 13-4), and have noted that this observation also applies to alkaline phosphatase activity at the lateral margins of the epithelial cells (Figure 13-5). Some metaplastic cells may lack the normal complement of intestinal enzymes. Kawachi et al. (9) found that sucrase activity may be limited to the junction of the antrum and the oxyntic mucosa when, in the same stomach, maltase activity may be present throughout the entire antrum. Nakahara (10) observed similar differences between parts of the stomach showing alkaline phosphatase and leucine aminopeptidase activity. These differences in the distribution of enzymes are matched by differences in the distribution of Paneth cells and mucous substances, and form the basis of the separation of intestinal metaplasia into complete and incomplete types by Matsukura et al. (12). The sucrase of the metaplastic mucosa may differ from that of the small intestine in one other respect. Kurisu et al. (13)

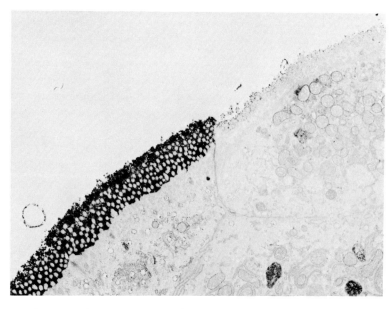

Figure 13-4.   Note the juxtaposition of alkaline phosphatase-positive and -negative metaplastic cells. Stained for alkaline phosphatase. × 3,550.

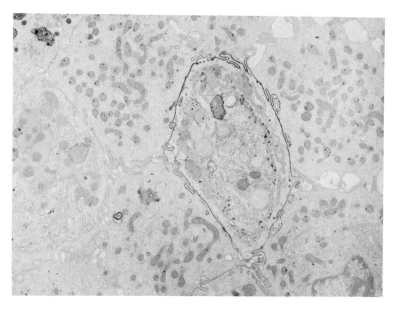

Figure 13-5.   The lateral plasma membrane of a metaplastic cell is alkaline phosphatase positive, whereas that of other metaplastic cells is negative. Note a sharp transition between the positive and negative areas. Stained for alkaline phosphatase. × 3,500.

have shown that sucrase from the metaplastic mucosa may lack the antigenic sugar moiety associated with blood group activity.

Mucus Histochemistry

The mucous substances of the metaplastic gastric mucosa may or may not resemble those of the small gut (12, 14). The mucus in jejunal goblet cells is consistently stained with alcian blue, but in metaplastic gastric mucosa the goblets of some cells may stain with high-iron diamine instead. Matsukura et al. (12) noted that iron diamine-positive cells are most likely to be found in metaplastic glands that lack Paneth cells and produce no alkaline phosphatase. Lastly, we have found that some metaplastic cells are hybrids, containing both mucous vacuoles and Paneth cell granules when seen by ultrastructure (Figure 13-6).

Cilia and Microvilli

Approximately 10 percent of stomachs showing intestinal metaplasia contain cysts lined by ciliated, iron diamine-positive cells. Cilia are not normally found in any part of the human gastrointestinal tract, and those in the stomach are clearly dysplastic. The dysplasia is mani-

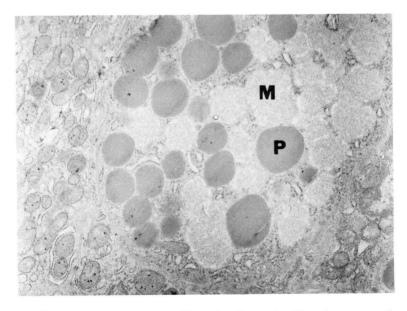

Figure 13-6.   Note the coexistence of Paneth cell granules (P) and mucous cell granules (M) in a single cell. × 3,500.

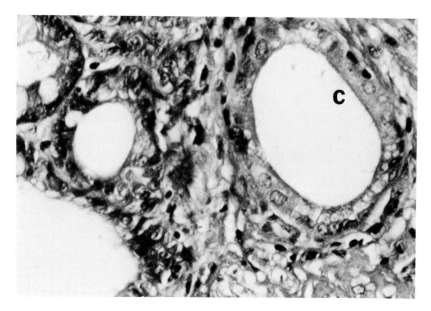

Figure 13-7.   A benign metaplastic gland showing ciliated cells (C). Trichrome stain. × 850.

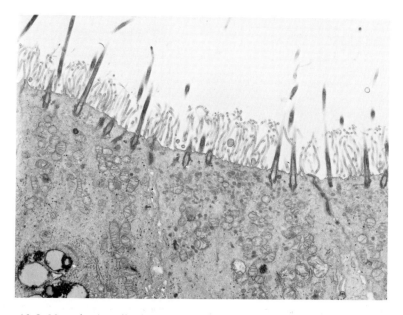

Figure 13-8. Metaplastic cells showing cilia and long-branching microvilli. × 3,500.

fest by variations from the usual 9:2 ratio of peripheral and central microtubules (Figures 13-7 to 13-9). The ciliated cells also have branching, "bushy" microvilli that are much longer than the microvilli of the small bowel (Figure 13-8). Such microvilli are not normally found in the gastrointestinal tract, but may be found in the epididymis (15) and in mesotheliomas (16).

Paneth Cells

Paneth cells are found in all of the crypts of the small intestinal mucosa, but not in all of the intestinalized glands of the stomach. Areas of intestinal metaplasia at the junction of the antral and oxyntic segments of the gastric mucosa are most likely to contain Paneth cells, and metaplastic glands in the distal antrum are less likely to contain them. In addition to the presence of Paneth-mucous cell hybrids, two other characteristics of these cells suggest that they are different from similar cells in the small bowel: The metaplastic Paneth cells are frequently quite superficial in location, especially those that accompany severe atypia; and [3H]TdR labeling has indicated that many of the metaplastic Paneth cells, unlike those of the small bowel, show active DNA synthesis.

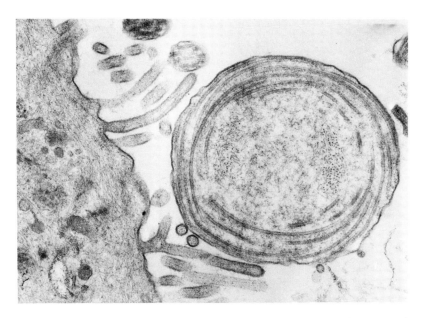

Figure 13-9.   A compound cilium with peripherally and concentrically arranged microtubules and central microfilaments. Note also a branching microvillus. × 30,500.

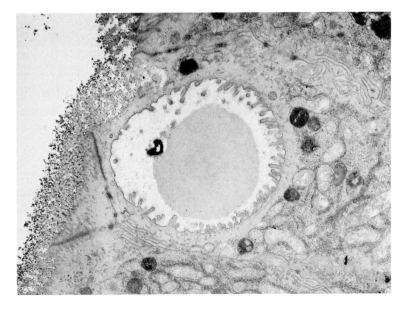

Figure 13-10.   Note an intracytoplasmic cyst with microvilli. ×3,500.

Intracytoplasmic Cysts

The cells of malignant epithelial neoplasms not infrequently contain intracytoplasmic cysts lined by microvilli, such as are normally present only on the luminal surfaces of normal epithelial cells. We have also found such cysts in the metaplastic epithelium (Figure 13-10) and consider such cells to be dysplastic.

DISCUSSION

In spite of their structural and functional similarities, the mucosa of the small intestine and the intestinalized gastric mucosa are clearly different tissues. Site-dependent variations in mucus and enzyme production suggest that the metaplastic epithelial cells are mutants, but other differences are more clearly dysplastic. These include the presence of cilia and "bushy" microvilli, hybrid mucous-Paneth cells, and intracytoplasmic cysts lined by microvilli. Intestinal metaplasia, therefore, may be a step in the development of at least some gastric carcinomas. This conclusion is supported by the frequent occurrence of early tumors in areas of metaplasia, the presence of intestinal metaplasia in the stomachs of animals given carcinogens at doses lower than necessary to induce cancer, and the epidemiologic association of metaplasia and cancer in high-risk populations. It should be noted, however, that intestinal metaplasia does not always precede cancer in humans or experimental animals, and hence is not an obligatory step in this process.

As seen by light microscopy, the intestinalized mucosa may show none of the attributes that characterize dysplasia (e.g., cellular and nuclear pleomorphism, loss of nuclear basal polarity, nuclear hyperchromatism, abnormal mitotic figures, etc.); yet this same mucosa may show ultrastructural changes that are clearly dysplastic. With some justice, this might be termed "occult dysplasia." Its biologic importance is in the eye of the beholder. Epidemiologic pathologists would appear to be justified in accepting its presence as evidence of exposure to one or more mutagenic events. On the other hand, surgical pathologists can assure their patients that it constitutes no immediate threat to their health or survival. If the process is sufficiently extensive to be associated with decreased acid production, patients should probably be warned that they are at increased risk for developing gastric carcinoma and that they should be reexamined at 3- to 5-year intervals so as to identify cancer at an early stage if it were to develop.

REFERENCES

1. Correa, P., Cuello, C., and Duque, E. Carcinoma and intestinal metaplasia of the stomach in Colombian immigrants. *J. Natl. Cancer Inst.* 44 (1970):297–306.
2. Stemmermann, G. N., Haenszel, W., and Locke, F. Epidemiologic pathology of gastric ulcer and gastric carcinoma among Japanese in Hawaii. *J. Natl. Cancer Inst.* 58 (1977):13–20.
3. Matsukura, N., Kawachi, T., Sugimura, T., Nakadate, M., and Hirota, T. Induction of intestinal metaplasia and carcinoma in the glandular stomach of rats by N-alkyl-N'-nitro-N-nitrosoguanidine. *Gann* 70 (1979):181–185.
4. Watanabe, H. Experimentally induced intestinal metaplasia in Wistar rats by x-ray irradiation. *Gastroenterology* 75 (1978):796–799.
5. Nakamura, K., Sugano, H., and Takagi, K. Carcinoma of the stomach in its incipient phase: Its histogenesis and histological appearances. *Gann* 59 (1968): 251–258.
6. Shimosato, Y., Tanaka, N., Kogure, K., Fujimura, S., Kawachi, T., and Sugimura, T. Histopathology of tumors of canine alimentary tract produced by N-methyl-N'-nitro-N-nitrosoguanidine, with particular reference to gastric cancer. *J. Natl. Cancer Inst.* 47 (1971):1053–1070.
7. Oohara, T., Tohma, H., Takezoe, K., Okawa, S., Johjima, Y., Asakura, R., Aono, G., and Kurosaka, H. Minute gastric carcinomas less than 5 mm in diameter. *Cancer* 50 (1982):801–810.
8. Stemmermann, G. N., and Hayashi, T. Intestinal metaplasia of the gastric mucosa: A gross and microscopic study of its distribution in various disease states. *J. Natl. Cancer Inst.* 41 (1968):627–634.

9. Kawachi, T., Kogure, K., Tanaka, N., Tokunaga, A., Sugimura, T., Koyama, T., Kanasugi, K., Hirota, T., and Sano, R. Studies of intestinal metaplasia in the gastric mucosa by the detection of disaccharidases with "Tes-Tape." *J. Natl. Cancer Inst.* 53 (1974):19–30.

10. Nakahara, K. Special features of intestinal metaplasia and its relation to early gastric cancer in man: Observations by method in which leucine aminopeptidase activity is used. *J. Natl. Cancer Inst.* 61 (1978):693–702.

11. Kumagae, Y. Enzyme histochemical studies of intestinal metaplasia in human stomach with special reference to electron microscopy [Japanese]. *Jpn. Soc. Dig. Sys.* 76 (1979):17–30.

12. Matsukura, N., Suzuki, K., Kawachi, T., Aoyagi, M., Sugimura, T., Kitaoka, H., Numajiri, H., Shirota, A., Itabashi, M., and Hirota, T. Distribution of marker enzymes and mucin in intestinal metaplasia of the stomach and relation of complete and incomplete types of metaplasia to minute gastric cancer. *J. Natl. Cancer Inst.* 65 (1980):231–236.

13. Kurisu, M., Numanyu, N., Kawachi, T., and Sugimura, T. Blood group activity of human sucrase from intestinal metaplasia. *J. Biol. Chem.* 252 (1977):3277–3280.

14. Stemmermann, G. N. Comparative study of histochemical patterns in non-neoplastic and neoplastic gastric epithelium: A study of Japanese in Hawaii. *J. Natl. Cancer Inst.* 39 (1967):375–382.

15. Fawcett, D. W. *The Cell*, 2nd ed., pp. 598–599. Philadelphia: W. B. Saunders, 1981.

16. Wang, N.-S. Electron microscopy in the diagnosis of mesothelioma. *Cancer* 31 (1973):1046–1054.

14 ROLE OF INTESTINAL METAPLASIA IN THE HISTOGENESIS OF GASTRIC CANCER

J. R. Jass

THE ORIGIN AND NATURE OF INTESTINAL METAPLASIA

The term "metaplasia" means the replacement of one adult tissue by another. Intestinal metaplasia of the stomach is generally interpreted as the substitution of gastric mucosa by an epithelium of the small intestinal type. It is also understood that intestinal metaplasia is an acquired heterotopia, developing on the basis of chronic gastritis (1). Some appreciation of the structure of normal small intestine helps one to understand the nature of intestinal metaplasia. The small intestinal mucosa may be divided into an upper villous compartment and a lower crypt compartment. The villi are lined by goblet cells and brightly eosinophilic columnar cells with a refractile brush border. The ratio of goblet cells to absorptive cells increases as one moves distally. The crypts are lined by columnar cells that lack a well-developed brush border and show secretory activity (2). These secretory columnar cells are the precursors of the mature absorptive cells lining the villi. The switch from secretory to absorptive activity occurs quite suddenly as the cells enter the villous compartment. Paneth cells occupy the crypt base.

The above features are all reproduced in intestinal metaplasia, except that the villi may be poorly developed and the separation of crypt and villous compartments may not be clear-cut (Figure 14-1). However, metaplastic epithelium may not necessarily show complete intestinal differentiation. In particular, the switch from secretory to absorptive function may either not take place or be only partially achieved (3). Intestinal metaplasia may therefore be divided according to whether intestinal differentiation is complete or incomplete (4–7). Incomplete intestinal metaplasia is illustrated in Figure 14-2.

The goblet cells of complete intestinal metaplasia secrete sialomucins like those of normal small intestine and little if any sulfomucin (Figure 14-3). On the other hand, some examples of incomplete intestinal metaplasia may secrete large amounts of sulfomucin. This property is evidenced by the columnar cell population in particular (Figure 14-4). The mucous cells of normal gastric epithelium secrete a neutral mucosubstance. An exception are the partially differentiated crypt base cells, which secrete small amounts of acid mucus. This appears to

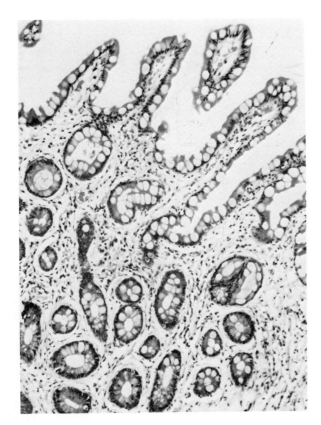

Figure 14-1.   Complete intestinal metaplasia. Villi are partially formed and lined by goblet cells and absorptive columnar cells. H&E stain. × 80.

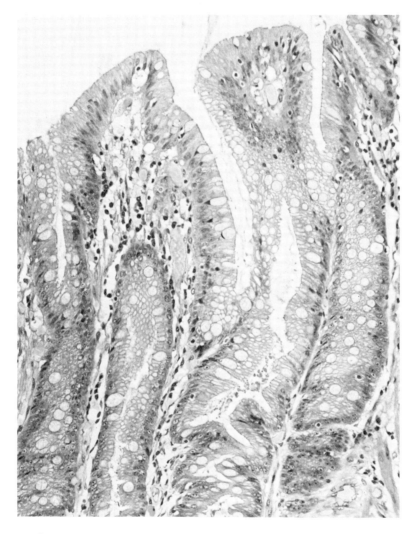

Figure 14-2.   Incomplete intestinal metaplasia. The mucosa is thickened and the crypts are branched and tortuous. The ratio of columnar to goblet cells is increased, and the columnar cells contain an apical, mucin-filled vesicle. The cells are notably tall and crowded. The goblet cells vary in size and some appear dislocated. The nuclei are enlarged slightly and are vesicular with prominent nucleoli. Paneth cells and mature enterocytes cannot be discerned. This example of incomplete intestinal metaplasia would be regarded as showing low-grade dysplasia. An "intestinal"-type carcinoma (not shown) occurred nearby. H&E stain. × 80.

include sulfomucin (8, 9). The sulfomucin-secreting columnar cells of incomplete intestinal metaplasia are probably close relatives of these partially differentiated crypt base cells.

(Text continues on page 172)

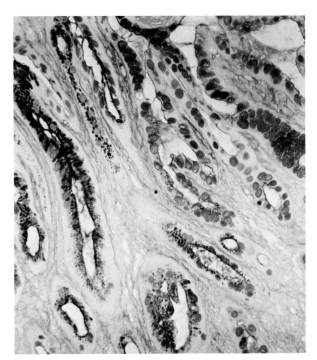

Figure 14-3.   The field shows complete intestinal metaplasia on the right and incomplete intestinal metaplasia on the left. The goblet cells in both areas secrete sialomucins (gray). The intervening columnar cells of incomplete intestinal metaplasia secrete sulfomucin (black). An adenoma (not shown) adjoined the field of incomplete intestinal metaplasia. HID/AB stain. × 80.

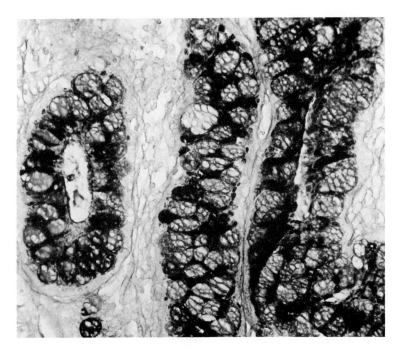

Figure 14-4.   High-power field of incomplete intestinal metaplasia. The goblet cells secrete sialomucins (gray) and the crowded intervening columnar cells secrete sulfomucins (black). HID/AB stain. × 288.

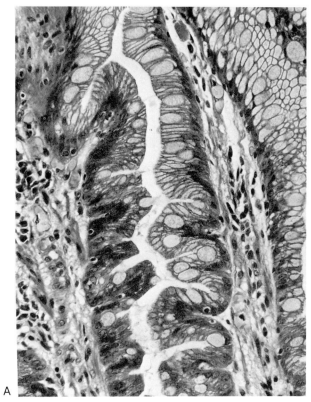

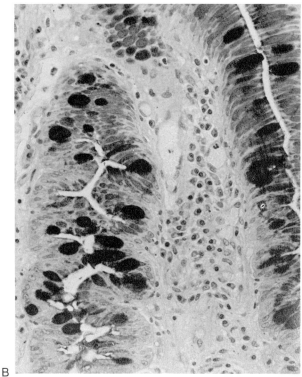

Figure 14-5. A: In-
complete intestinal
metaplasia. The goblet
cells are scattered
among tall, mucin-
filled columnar cells.
An intestinal-type
carcinoma (not shown)
occurred nearby. H&E
stain. × 288. B: Serial
section of (A). Both
the columnar and
goblet cells secrete
acid mucus. The darker
goblet cells are more
PAS positive than the
columnar cells. The
former secrete sialomu-
cins and the latter sul-
fomucins. AB/diastase
PAS stain. × 288.

HISTOLOGICAL IDENTIFICATION OF INCOMPLETE
INTESTINAL METAPLASIA

Incomplete intestinal metaplasia is recognized in histological sections by the presence of goblet cells and columnar mucous cells and the apparent absence of mature absorptive cells and Paneth cells. However, in certain circumstances its identification may prove difficult. In some instances the columnar cells secrete abundant mucus and the small numbers of goblet cells are relatively inconspicuous. Such epithelium could on superficial inspection be interpreted as the normal gastric type (Figure 14-5A, B). In contrast, the columnar cells may se crete minimal amounts of mucus and thereby resemble absorptive cells. Such mucosa may be incorrectly labeled as complete intestinal metaplasia (Figure 14-6). The presence of severe regenerative change may make the separation of complete and incomplete intestinal meta-

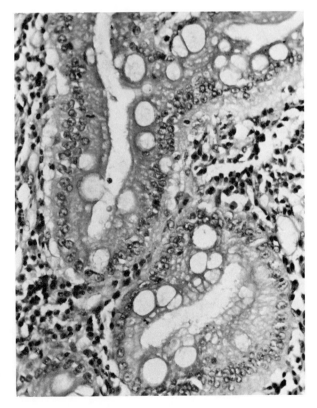

Figure 14-6. Incomplete intestinal metaplasia in which the columnar cells secrete minimal amounts of mucus (sulfomucin). The goblet cells are relatively sparse, vary in size, and appear dislocated. The nuclei are enlarged, vesicular, and show focal loss of polarity. This field is regarded as showing low-grade dysplasia. An intramucosal carcinoma (not shown) arose 1 centimeter from this field. H&E stain. × 288.

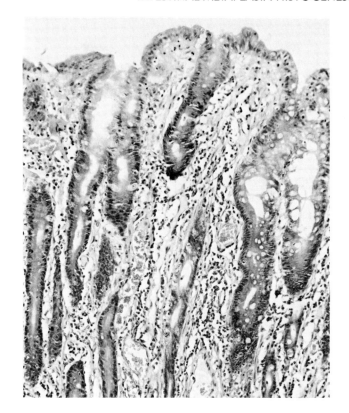

Figure 14-7. Severe regenerative change within incomplete intestinal metaplasia. The metaplastic nature of this field together with the secretion of sulfomucin were confirmed with the HID/AB technique (not shown). Goblet cells can, in fact, be easily recognized in the crypts to the right. This field resembles a lesion termed "basal cell proliferation," which occurs in chronic ulcerative colitis. This would be regarded as a form of low-grade dysplasia. An intestinal-type carcinoma (not shown) occurred nearby. H&E stain. × 80.

plasia difficult (Figure 14-7). These problems may be circumvented by staining sections routinely with alcian blue (pH 2.5)/diastase periodic acid-Schiff stain. The goblet cells are then easily identified by their secretion of acid mucus (blue), whereas the columnar cells stain blue-purple or red, depending on the proportions of neutral and acid mucus. If they stain purple or blue, this usually indicates the secretion of sulfomucin. This can be confirmed with the high-iron diamine/alcian blue technique (10), which stains sulfomucins brown and sialomucins blue.

RELATION BETWEEN SULFOMUCIN-POSITIVE INTESTINAL METAPLASIA AND GASTRIC CANCER

Marked secretion of sulfomucin characterizes incomplete rather than complete intestinal metaplasia. However, not all examples of incomplete intestinal metaplasia secrete sulfomucin. Variants of incomplete intestinal metaplasia secreting sulfomucin will henceforth be termed "S-Pos." A number of studies have demonstrated an association between S-Pos intestinal metaplasia and gastric carcinoma (7, 11–14). The material discussed here included 30 carcinomas and 25 benign specimens showing extensive intestinal metaplasia (6). S-Pos intestinal metaplasia was found in 17 (57 percent) of the cancer specimens but in only 2 (8 percent) of the benign specimens. In a comparable study, 49 percent of the cancerous specimens included S-Pos intestinal metaplasia, whereas only 5 percent of the benign, extensively intestinalized specimens revealed this lesion (14). These figures indicate that within the entity of intestinal metaplasia, S-Pos variants show a selective association with gastric carcinoma.

The occurrence of S-Pos intestinal metaplasia was investigated in an endoscopic survey of a large Finnish population (13). Intestinal metaplasia of any type was detected in 61 patients with gastric cancer and in a total of 316 patients with no malignancy. (These authors graded sulfomucin secretion into weak and strong. The following figures are based on the strong reaction only). Thirty-one percent of malignant cases showed S-Pos intestinal metaplasia, whereas only 6 percent of the benign cases revealed this lesion. S-Pos intestinal metaplasia would therefore also appear to be a selective marker of gastric carcinoma in endoscopic biopsy material. Indeed, the low incidence of false positives makes the test a viable one for screening purposes. Unfortunately, the sensitivity is low, as indicated by the high proportion of false negatives.

Although S-Pos intestinal metaplasia shows a selective association with gastric carcinoma, this does not necessarily prove that the lesion has a cancerous potential over and above other epithelial types. However, a number of observations suggest that S-Pos intestinal metaplasia may play an important role in the histogenesis of gastric carcinoma. Gastric carcinoma has been classified into two histogenic types. The "intestinal" type is thought to arise within intestinal metaplasia and the "diffuse" type in normal gastric mucosa. This certainly appears to be the case at a statistical level, though individual exceptions may of course be found (15). S-Pos intestinal metaplasia shows a significant association with intestinal- as opposed to diffuse-type carcinomas (6).

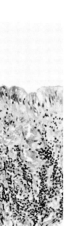
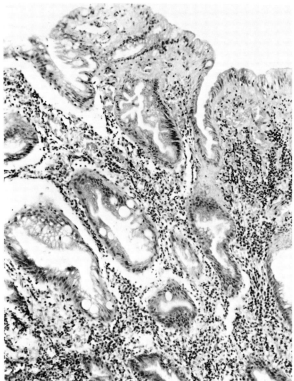

Figure 14-8.
Carcinoma (*lower left*)
arising in incomplete
intestinal metaplasia.
The columnar cells
of the metaplastic
epithelium do not
show obvious mucus
secretion in this
section. However, the
HID/AB technique (not
shown) demonstrated
intense staining for
sulfomucin in the cell
apex. The metaplastic
crypts show marked
serration, reminiscent
of the metaplastic
polyp of the colorec-
tum. H&E stain. × 80.

Patients with S-Pos intestinal metaplasia are likely to be older than pa-tients with S-Neg (13). Intestinal-type carcinomas show a similar pre-dilection for the elderly (15). S-Pos intestinal metaplasia is frequently present in the immediate vicinity of intestinal-type carcinomas (6; Fig-ure 14-8). The mucin profiles of S-Pos intestinal metaplasia and intesti-nal-type carcinoma are similar, with sulfomucins predominating (16–18). These findings suggest either that S-Pos intestinal metaplasia is the precursor of intestinal-type carcinoma or that the lesions share an etiological factor.

An inquiry into the relationship between intestinal metaplasia and gastric dysplasia suggests that S-Pos intestinal metaplasia is in fact precancerous (19). It is possible to demonstrate a continuum through dysplasia to carcinoma. S-Pos intestinal metaplasia shows a number of atypical features in itself. These include its incomplete intestinal dif-ferentiation, with the absence of Paneth and mature absorptive cells.

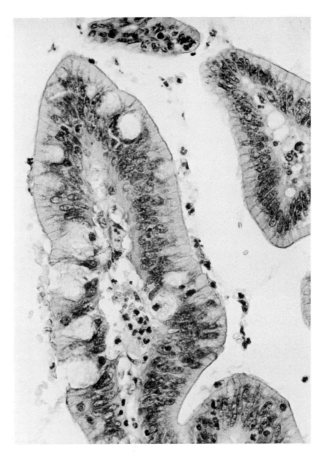

Figure 14-9.   Adenomatous epithelium showing incomplete intestinal differentiation. The goblet cells are bordered by columnar mucous cells. This suggests that incomplete intestinal metaplasia and epithelial dysplasia may form a continuum. H&E stain. × 360.

The crypts are often excessively tall (occupying a thickened mucosa) and show architectural abnormalities including irregular branching, budding, cyst formation, and marked tortuosity. The lining cells are taller and more crowded than their counterparts within complete intestinal metaplasia. Nuclei are enlarged, rounded, and vesicular. These features are illustrated in Figures 14-2, 14-5A, and 14-6. Adenomas—themselves associated with a significant cancerous risk—have been observed to arise in S-Pos intestinal metaplasia (20) and may resemble it in spite of their loss of differentiation (Figure 14-9).

CLINICAL IMPLICATIONS OF SULFOMUCIN-POSITIVE INTESTINAL METAPLASIA

The discovery of S-Pos intestinal metaplasia in a gastric biopsy is usually indicative of an accompanying carcinoma (13). In cases where no tumor is identified, precise guidelines on management cannot be given until the natural history of S-Pos intestinal metaplasia is clarified. Follow-up studies will reveal the magnitude of risk in time. Meanwhile, annual endoscopic follow-up surveillance is advocated. Favorable subjects for endoscopic screening would be inhabitants of high-risk areas or persons with precancerous conditions such as pernicious anemia and gastric stumps. Particular precancerous conditions may not necessarily provide the appropriate environment for histogenic pathways involving S-Pos intestinal metaplasia. S-Pos intestinal metaplasia is found with increased frequency in patients with pernicious anemia (13), but has not yet been described in gastric stumps. Furthermore, although the studies cited above showed S-Pos intestinal metaplasia to be a selective marker of gastric cancer, this might not necessarily apply to all populations.

ACKNOWLEDGMENTS

I am grateful to Mr. P. Ahern of the Central Middlesex Hospital, London, for photographic help.

REFERENCES

1. Magnus, H. A. Observations on the presence of intestinal epithelium in the gastric mucosa. *J. Pathol. Bacteriol.* 44 (1937):389–397.
2. Trier, J. S. Studies on small intestinal crypt epithelium. II. Evidence for and mechanisms of secretory activity by undifferentiated crypt cells of the human small intestine. *Gastroenterology* 58 (1964):444–461.
3. Ming, S.-C. Goldman, H., and Freiman, D. G. Intestinal metaplasia and histogenesis of carcinoma of the human stomach. *Cancer* 20 (1967):1418–1429.
4. Iida, F., Murata, F., and Nagata, T. Histochemical studies of mucosubstances in metaplastic epithelium of the stomach with special reference to the development of intestinal metaplasia. *Histochem. J.* 56 (1978):229–237.
5. Nakahara, K. Special features of intestinal metaplasia and its relation to early gastric carcinoma in man. Observation by a method in which leucine aminopeptidase activity is used. *J. Natl. Cancer Inst.* 61 (1978):693–701.
6. Jass, J. R. Role of intestinal metaplasia in the histogenesis of gastric carcinoma. *J. Clin. Pathol.* 33 (1980):801–810.

7. Matsukura, N., Suzuki, K., Kawachi, T., Aoyagi, M., Sugimura, T., Kitaoka, H., Numajiri, H., Shirota, A., Itabashi, M., and Hirota, T. Distribution of marker enzymes and mucin in intestinal metaplasia in human stomachs and relation of complete and incomplete types of metaplasia to minute gastric carcinomas. *J. Natl. Cancer Inst.* 65 (1980):231–240.

8. Goldman, H., and Ming, S. -C. Mucins in normal and neoplastic gastrointestinal epithelium. *Arch. Pathol.* 85 (1968):580–586.

9. Montero, C., and Segura, D. I. Retrospective histochemical study of mucosubstances in adenocarcinomas of the gastrointestinal tract. *Histopathology* 4 (1980):281–292.

10. Spicer, S. S. Diamine methods for differentiating mucosubstances histochemically. *J. Histochem. Cytochem.* 13 (1965):211–234.

11. Heilman, K. L., and Höpker, W. W. Loss of differentiation in intestinal metaplasia in cancerous stomachs. A comparative morphologic study. *Pathol. Res. Pract.* 164 (1979):249–258.

12. Jass, J. R., and Filipe, M. I. A variant of intestinal metaplasia associated with gastric carcinoma. A histochemical study. *Histopathology* 3 (1979):191–199.

13. Sipponen, P., Seppälä, K., Varis, K., Hjelt, L., Ihamaki, T., Kekki, M., and Siurala, M. Intestinal metaplasia with colonic-type sulphomucins in the gastric mucosa; its association with gastric carcinoma. *Acta Pathol. Microbiol. Scand. (A)* 88 (1980):217–224.

14. Wells, M., Stewart, M., and Dixon, M. F. Mucin histochemistry of gastric intestinal metaplasia [Abstract]. *J. Pathol.* 138 (1982):70.

15. Laurén, P. The two main histological types of gastric carcinoma: Diffuse and so-called intestinal type carcinoma. *Acta Pathol. Microbiol. Scand.* 64 (1965):31–49.

16. Gad, A. A histochemical study of human alimentary tract mucosubstances in health and disease. I. Normal and tumour. *Br. J. Cancer* 23 (1969):52–63.

17. Laurén, P., and Sorvari, T. Mucin histochemistry in diffuse and intestinal type carcinoma. *Scand. J. Clin. Invest. (Suppl.)* 108 (1969):70.

18. Jass, J. R., and Filipe, M. I. The mucin profiles of normal gastric mucosa, intestinal metaplasia and its variants and gastric carcinoma. *Histochem. J.* 13 (1981):931–939.

19. Jass, J. R. A classification of gastric dysplasia. *Histopathology* 7 (1983):181–193.

20. Jass, J. R., and Filipe, M. I. Sulphomucins and precancerous lesions of the human stomach. *Histopathology* 4 (1980):271–279.

15 SIGNIFICANCE OF INTESTINAL METAPLASIA AS A PRECANCEROUS CONDITION OF THE STOMACH

T. Hirota, T. Okada, M. Itabashi,
H. Yoshida, N. Matsukura, H. Kitaoka,
and T. Hirayama

There have been many reports concerning the histogenesis of gastric cancer. Some authors have reported a certain relationship between carcinoma and intestinal metaplasia (1–3). Nakamura et al. (3) concluded from their data that well-differentiated adenocarcinoma arose in the metaplastic mucosa and that poorly differentiated adenocarcinoma occurred in the nonmetaplastic mucosa.

In order to clarify the significance of intestinal metaplasia as a precancerous lesion, we reviewed histologically 650 early gastric cancers, 62 small gastric carcinomas, 52 adenomas, and 149 hyperplastic polyps in relation to metaplastic mucosa. This chapter is a summary of the study.

RELATIONSHIP BETWEEN EARLY GASTRIC CANCER AND INTESTINAL METAPLASIA

The materials studied were 650 early gastric cancers from 600 cases that were surgically resected at the National Cancer Center Hospital in Tokyo, Japan, from 1962 to 1975. The sections were cut parallel to the lesser curvature and included the whole area of cancerous lesion and the surrounding mucosa to allow an examination of the distribution of gastritis. The location of the cancer and the distribution of the mucosa with intestinal metaplasia were schematically reconstructed on a picture of each stomach in order to examine the spatial relationship between carcinoma and metaplastic mucosa.

According to the general rules for gastric cancer study in surgery and pathology developed by the Japanese Research Society for Gastric Cancer (4), carcinoma was classified as follows: papillary adenocarcinoma; tubular adenocarcinoma; poorly differentiated adenocarcinoma; and mucocellular adenocarcinoma (including muconodular adenocarcinoma in this chapter). The former two types will be referred to as "differentiated adenocarcinoma," and the latter two as "undifferentiated adenocarcinoma."

We also classified the materials into four groups (see Table 15-1) for the study of the spatial relation of carcinoma to the distribution of metaplastic mucosa as follows: Group I (69 lesions) was composed of gastric cancers that were completely surrounded by mucosa with intestinal metaplasia. In Group II (482 lesions) the cancer was located in continuity with, but not completely surrounded by, the area of intestinal metaplasia. In Group III (90 lesions) the cancer was located inside

Table 15-1. Relations between Intestinal Metaplasia and Histological Types of Gastric Cancer (Early Gastric Cancer, 600 Cases, 650 Lesions)

| | Histological Types | | |
	Differentiated	Undifferentiated	Total
Group I	60	9	69
	(87.0)	(13.0)	(100)
Group II	257	225	482
	(53.3)	(46.7)	(100)
Group III	13	77	90
	(14.4)	(85.6)	(100)
Group IV	5	4	9
	(55.6)	(44.5)	(100)
Total	335	315	650
	(51.5)	(48.5)	(100)

Numbers in parentheses are percentages.

Table 15-2. Relations between Histological Types of Gastric Cancer and
Age of Patients (Early Gastric Cancer, 650 Lesions)

	Histological Types				
	Differentiated		Undifferentiated		
			Poorly		
Age (years)	Papillary Adeno-carcinoma	Tubular Adeno-carcinoma	Differentiated Adeno-carcinoma	Mucocellular Adeno-carcinoma	Total
≤29	—	1	1	7	9
30–39	1	10	16	41	68
40–49	7	30	20	75	132
50–59	20	66	30	53	169
≥60	58	142	34	38	272
Total	86	249	101	214	650

the mucosa without intestinal metaplasia. Cancers in Group IV were located in areas of verrucous gastritis (9 lesions).

The age of the patients and the histological types of cancer are shown in Table 15-2. Both papillary and tubular adenocarcinomas were more frequently seen in the older age group (older than 50 years); over one-half of the patients were in their seventh decade. In contrast, undifferentiated adenocarcinoma was relatively frequent in patients in their fifth decade.

The frequency and age distribution of the various histological types of cancers in Group I are listed Table 15-3. The data show that the frequency of differentiated adenocarcinoma in each decade increased with increasing age. The same tendency was observed in

Table 15-3. Relations between Histological Types of Gastric Cancer and
Age of Patients (Group I, 69 Lesions)

	Histological Types				
	Differentiated		Undifferentiated		
			Poorly		
Age (years)	Papillary Adeno-carcinoma	Tubular Adeno-carcinoma	Differentiated Adeno-carcinoma	Mucocellular Adeno-carcinoma	Total
≤29	0	0	0	0	0
30–39	0	0	0	0	0
40–49	2	0	2	1	5
50–59	1	8	2	0	11
≥60	14	35	3	1	53
Total	17	43	7	2	69

Table 15-4. Relations between Histological Types of Gastric Cancer and
Age of Patients (Group II, 491 Lesions)

	Histological Types				
	Differentiated		Undifferentiated		
			Poorly		
Age (years)	Papillary Adeno-carcinoma	Tubular Adeno-carcinoma	Differentiated Adeno-carcinoma	Mucocellular Adeno-carcinoma	Total
≤29	0	1	0	3	4
30–39	1	6	11	23	41
40–49	5	29	15	50	99
50–59	17	56	24	43	140
≥60	44	103	29	31	207
Total	67	195	79	150	491

Groups II and III (Tables 15-4 and 15-5). Tables 15-6 and 15-7 show the relation between the histological types of cancer with the age of the patients and with ulceration of the cancerous lesion. Cancers with ulceration or with ulcer scars within the cancerous lesion were more frequent in undifferentiated adenocarcinoma. On the other hand, 195 of 215 lesions with no ulceration were differentiated adenocarcinoma. Undifferentiated adenocarcinoma in nonulcerative-type cancer was found in only a small number of cases (20 of 215).

Relative-to-identified-distribution analysis (5; RIDIT) was used to confirm the statistical significance of the relation between the histological types of cancer and three factors—intestinal metaplasia, age,

Table 15-5. Relations between Histological Types of Gastric Cancer and
Age of Patients (Group III, 90 Lesions)

	Histological Types				
	Differentiated		Undifferentiated		
			Poorly		
Age (years)	Papillary Adeno-carcinoma	Tubular Adeno-carcinoma	Differentiated Adeno-carcinoma	Mucocellular Adeno-carcinoma	Total
≤29	0	0	1	4	5
30–39	0	4	5	18	27
40–49	0	1	3	24	28
50–59	2	2	4	10	18
≥60	1	3	2	6	12
Total	3	10	15	62	90

Table 15-6. Relations between Histological Types of Gastric Cancer and Age of Patients (Ulcerated-Type Early Gastric Cancer, 435 Lesions)

| | Histological Types | | | | |
| | Differentiated | | Undifferentiated | | |
Age (years)	Papillary Adeno-carcinoma	Tubular Adeno-carcinoma	Poorly Differ-entiated Ade-nocarcinoma	Mucocellular Adeno-carcinoma	Total
≤29	0	0	1	7	8
30–39	0	8	15	39	62
40–49	0	20	17	75	112
50–59	2	45	25	52	124
≥60	3	62	27	37	129
Total	5	135	85	210	435

and ulceration. In Figure 15-1 the vertical axis indicates the degree of differentiation of the cancer: 0.50 is the average RIDIT of the differentiation range of the cancer. Each of the above three factors is represented along the horizontal axis. The heavy black line indicates a rough RIDIT, and the light dashed line is the standard RIDIT, which stands for the relation between the degree of differentiation of the cancer and each of three factors on the horizontal axis, independent of the influence of the other factors. RIDIT analysis led to the same conclusion mentioned above with regard to statistical significance and showed that each of the three factors has its own relation to the degree of differentiation of the cancer, independent of the influence of the other factors.

Table 15-7. Relations between Histological Types of Gastric Cancer and Age of Patients (Nonulcerated-Type Early Gastric Cancer, 215 Lesions)

| | Histological Types | | | | |
| | Differentiated | | Undifferentiated | | |
Age (years)	Papillary Adeno-carcinoma	Tubular Adeno-carcinoma	Poorly Differ-entiated Ade-nocarcinoma	Mucocellular Adeno-carcinoma	Total
≤29	0	1	0	0	1
30–39	1	2	1	2	6
40–49	7	10	3	0	20
50–59	18	21	5	1	45
≥60	56	79	7	1	143
Total	82	113	16	4	215

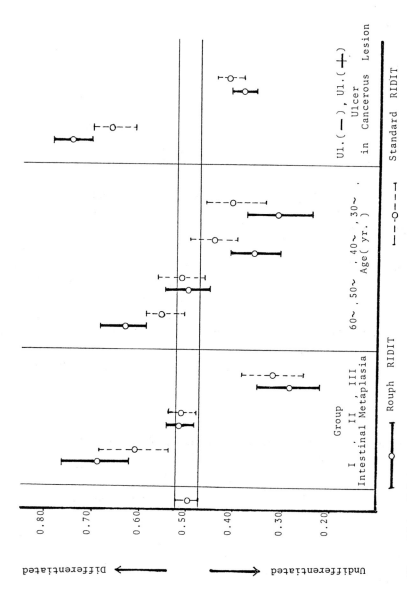

Figure 15-1. Relative-to-identified-distribution (RIDIT) analysis of relationship between histological dif-

In conclusion, gastric cancer frequently occurred at the margin of an area with intestinal metaplasia. Intestinal metaplasia appeared to be directly related to the presence of a differentiated adenocarcinoma. Other findings were that the degree of differentiation of the cancer increased with the age of the host and that nonulcerated adenocarcinoma often occurred among differentiated adenocarcinomas.

SPATIAL RELATION BETWEEN EARLY GASTRIC CANCER AND SUBTYPES OF INTESTINAL METAPLASIA

Intestinal metaplasia was classified histologically into two subtypes: complete and incomplete (6). The complete type was defined as

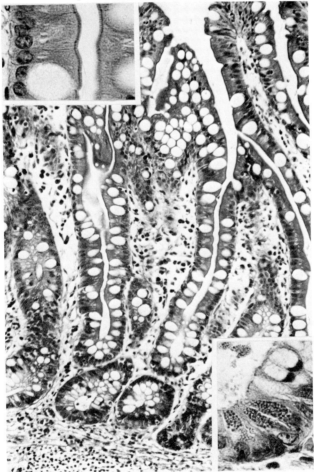

Figure 15-2.   Histology of the complete type of intestinal metaplasia of the stomach. Goblet cells, striated border, and Paneth cells are seen in the inset. H&E stain. × 100; × 400 (inset).

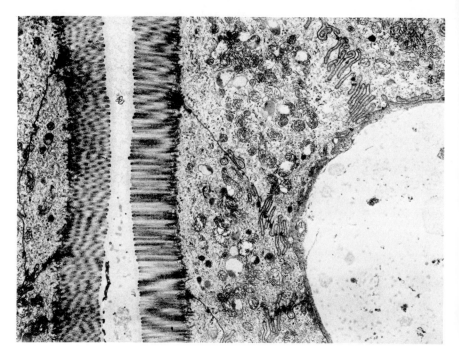

Figure 15-3.   Electron microscopic picture of complete-type metaplastic epithelium. Tall microvilli are arranged densely and regularly at the apical surface of the epthelium. × 5,500.

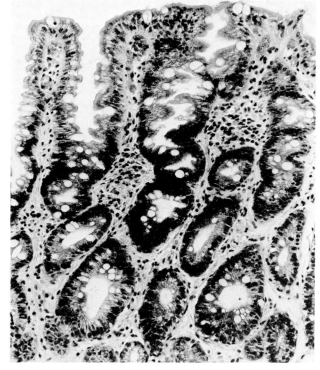

Figure 15-4.   Histology of the incomplete type of intestinal metaplasia of the stomach. Abnormal goblet cell population, absence of striated border, and Paneth cells are observed. H&E stain. × 100.

intestinal metaplasia with the presence of goblet cells, a striated epithelial border, and Paneth cells (Figures 15-2 and 15-3). The incomplete type was defined as intestinal metaplasia with the presence of goblet cells and/or a striated epithelial border and the absence of Paneth cells (Figures 15-4 and 15-5).

Histochemically and enzymologically, the complete-type intestinal metaplasia showed sucrase, trehalase, leucine aminopeptidase, and alkaline phosphatase activities and was negative for sulfomucin by high-iron diamine (HID) stain. The incomplete-type intestinal metaplasia showed sucrase and leucine aminopeptidase but no trehalase or alkaline phosphatase activities, and was sulfomucin positive by HID stain (Table 15-8).

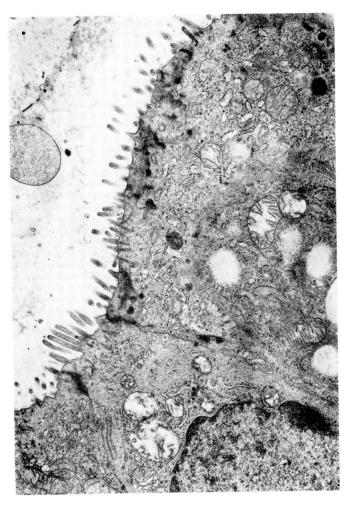

Figure 15-5.   Electron microscopic view of the incomplete-type metaplastic epithelium. Microvilli at the surface of the epithelium are scattered and irregularly arranged. The villi are not very high.   × 8,800.

Table 15-8. Morphological and Biochemical Characteristics of the
Complete and Incomplete Types of Intestinal Metaplasia

Markers	Intestinal Metaplasia	
	Complete Type	Incomplete Type
Paneth cells	+ +	−
Goblet cells	+ +	+ / + +
Striated border	+ + +	− / +
Sulfomucin	−	+ +
Sialomucin	+ +	− / +
Microvilli	+ + +	− / +
Sucrase	+	+
Trehalase	+	−
Leucine aminopeptidase	+	+
Alkaline phosphatase	+	−

− , Absent; + , present in small amount; + + , present in moderate amount; + + + , abundant.

It has been observed that the smaller the cancer, the better the mucosa is preserved (7). So, we reviewed 56 surgically resected stomachs with 62 minute or small carcinomas that were identified among 900 early gastric cancer cases during the last 16 years. The size of the small gastric cancer was less than 10 millimeters in the maximal diameter.

The age distribution of the 56 cases showed a peak in the seventh decade. The average age was 59.1 years, and the male-to-female ratio was 3.7. This average age was slightly older than that in the total early gastric cancer series of 900 cases. The male-to-female ratio was significantly higher than that of the total series. Thirty-five (56.5 percent) of the 62 lesions were found in the middle third, 26 (41.9 percent) in the lower third, and only 1 lesion in the upper third of the stomach. Differentiated adenocarcinoma showed the same localization as that of the total cases, except for a slightly higher frequency in the lower third. The superficial depressed type (IIc type) was the most frequent, according to the Japanese macroscopic-type classification for early gastric cancer (4). The depressed type (including IIc, IIc + III, and III) was found in 42 lesions (67.7 percent), the flat type (IIb) in 11 lesions (17.7 percent), and the elevated type (IIa and I) in 9 lesions (14.5 percent). The frequency of the IIb type in this series was remarkably higher than that of the series of 900 early gastric cancers.

The surrounding mucosa was histologically examined in an area of 9 square centimeters. There were 28 lesions whose surrounding mucosa showed intestinal metaplasia in more than 75 percent of the 9-square centimeter area. Twenty-six of 28 lesions were differentiated

Table 15-9. Relations between Minute and Small Early Gastric Cancers and Subtypes of Intestinal Metaplasia in the Adjacent Mucosa

Subtypes of Intestinal Metaplasia	0- to 5-mm cancer			0- to 10-mm cancer		
		Histology			Histology	
	No. of lesions	Differentiated Adenocarcinoma	Undifferentiated Adenocarcinoma	No. of lesions	Differentiated Adenocarcinoma	Undifferentiated Adenocarcinoma
Incomplete	10(43.5)	10(55.6)	0(0)	30(48.4)	27(62.8)	3(15.7)
Mixed	5(21.7)	4(22.2)	1(20.0)	7(11.3)	6(13.9)	1(5.3)
Complete	4(17.4)	3(16.7)	1(20.0)	13(21.0)	7(16.3)	6(31.6)
None	4(17.4)	1(5.6)	3(60.0)	12(19.3)	3(7.0)	9(47.4)
Total	23(100.0)	18(100.0)	5(100.0)	62(100.0)	43(100.0)	19(100.0)

Numbers in parentheses are percentages.

adenocarcinomas, and the other 2 were undifferentiated adenocarcinomas. In contrast, 14 lesions showed intestinal metaplasia in less than 25 percent of the 9-square centimeter surrounding mucosa. Only 2 of 14 lesions were differentiated adenocarcinoma, and the other 12 were undifferentiated.

The following study was done to clarify the spatial relationship between small carcinoma and the incomplete-type intestinal metaplasia. Table 15-9 shows the histologic findings of gastric mucosa directly adjacent to the cancerous lesion. Metaplastic glands of the incomplete type were found more frequently than both completely metaplastic and nonmetaplastic glands in the mucosa adjacent to the carcinoma. Especially in cases of differentiated adenocarcinoma, the tendency was remarkable. Undifferentiated adenocarcinoma was rarely seen adjacent to incomplete-type metaplastic mucosa.

These data suggest that carcinoma, especially differentiated adenocarcinoma, is likely to occur within mucosa of intestinal metaplasia, particularly the incomplete type.

SPATIAL RELATION BETWEEN SMALL ADENOMA OF THE STOMACH AND SUBTYPES OF INTESTINAL METAPLASIA

In order to study the background mucosa of gastric adenoma, the surrounding mucosa of the small lesions was examined histologically and histochemically. The specimens included 52 lesions from 45 surgically resected stomachs. The lesions were smaller than 1 centimeter in the maximal diameter.

Metaplastic mucosa was found in the adjacent area in 47 of 52 lesions. In metaplastic mucosa the incomplete type was most fre-

pattern	lesions	%	%
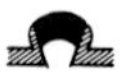 🔲	24	46.3	
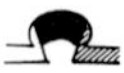 🔲	7	13.4	75.1
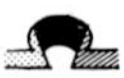 🔲	8	15.4	
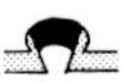 🔲	8	15.4	15.4
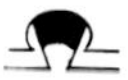 🔲	5	9.5	9.5
total	52	100	

incomplete type   complete type   none   **adenoma.**

Figure 15-6.   Distribution pattern of intestinal metaplasia around small adenoma (52 lesions) from 45 cases; 1962–79; National Cancer Center Hospital, Tokyo, Japan.

quently found more or less adjacent to the adenoma (31 of 52 lesions). Especially, 24 of 31 lesions were almost entirely surrounded by incomplete-type metaplastic mucosa. Complete-type metaplastic mucosa was found more or less adjacent to the lesion in 8 of 52 lesions. In contrast, nonmetaplastic mucosa was infrequently found adjacent to the lesions (5 of 52 lesions). Eight lesions were surrounded by both complete- and incomplete-type intestinal metaplasia (Figure 15-6).

As the cellular atypia of the adenoma increased, incomplete-type intestinal metaplasia adjacent to the adenoma increased in frequency. The six lesions that showed the most cellular atypia were surrounded by incomplete-type intestinal metaplasia. However, only 5 lesions were surrounded by incomplete-type intestinal metaplasia among 19 lesions showing mild cellular atypia.

In conclusion, these findings suggest that small adenoma has a closer relation with the incomplete type of intestinal metaplasia than with the complete type.

SPATIAL RELATION BETWEEN HYPERPLASTIC POLYP AND SUBTYPES OF INTESTINAL METAPLASIA

The background mucosa of hyperplastic polyps [also called regenerative polyps by Ming and Goldman (8)] were histologically examined in order to elucidate their relation to the incomplete type of metaplastic mucosa.

The materials consisted of 149 lesions from 90 cases that were surgically operated on from 1962 to 1970. The average age of the pa-

Type \ Size		~1.0 cm	1.1~2.0cm	2.1~cm	Total
Sessile		18 (12.1%)	2 (1.3%)	1 (0.7%)	21 (14.1%)
Short pedunculated		61 (40.9%)	8 (5.4%)	2 (1.3%)	71 (47.7%)
Pedunculated		29 (19.5%)	23 (15.4%)	5 (3.4%)	57 (38.2%)
Total		108	33	8	149 (100 %)

Figure 15-7.   Gross types and sizes of hyperplastic polyps (149 lesions).

tients was 55.2 years, and the male-to-female ratio was 0.96. Of the gross types of polyps, the short, pedunculated type was the most frequent (47.6 percent); most (94.6 percent) of the 141 polyps were less than 2 centimeters in diameter (Figure 15-7). About one-half of the 149 lesions were located in the lower third of the stomach.

The circumstantial factor of the hyperplastic polyp might be similar to that of verrucous gastritis, because 37.8 percent of the cases with the former had the latter. The surrounding mucosa was histologically examined in a width of 2 centimeters at each side of the polyp. Hyperplastic polyps were surrounded by complete-type, incomplete-type, or mixed-type metaplastic or nonmetaplastic mucosa. The frequencies were 30.9, 4.0, 21.5, and 43.6 percent, respectively (Figure 15-8).

		No. of lesions (%)	
Incomplete		6	(4.0)
Mixed		32	(21.5)
Complete		46	(30.9)
None		65	(43.6)
total		149	(100)

☐ hyperplastic polyp   ⊞ incomplete type
▨ complete type   ■ none

Figure 15-8.   Subtypes of intestinal metaplasia and hyperplastic polyps of the stomach (90 cases, 149 lesions).

Table 15-10. Relations between Subtypes of Intestinal Metaplasia and
Carcinoma, Adenoma, Hyperplastic Polyps, and Ulcers

Subtypes of Intestinal Metaplasia	Carcinoma < 1 cm		Adenoma < 1 cm		Hyperplastic Polyps		Benign Ulcers < 1 cm	
	No.	%	No.	%	No.	%	No.	%
Incomplete	30	48.4	31	59.7	6	4.0	7	9.3
Mixed	7	11.3	8	15.4	32	21.5	4	5.3
Complete	13	21.0	8	15.4	46	30.9	38	50.7
Nonmetaplastic	12	19.3	5	9.5	65	43.6	26	34.7
Total	62	100	52	100	149	100	75	100

These findings suggest that the regenerative hyperplastic lesion is not necessarily related to the incomplete-type metaplastic mucosa, in contrast to small carcinoma.

CONCLUSION

All the results from the present studies are summarized in Table 15-10. The findings suggest that differentiated adenocarcinoma and adenoma are spatially related to incomplete-type intestinal metaplasia, in contrast to nonneoplastic hyperplastic lesions.

It is strongly indicated that differentiated carcinoma and adenoma arise from metaplastic mucosa, especially of the incomplete type. However, it is still difficult to determine whether metaplastic mucosa is a real precancerous condition or a paracancerous condition that is produced under the same conditions that carcinoma is.

ACKNOWLEDGMENTS

The authors are greatly indebted to Dr. Y. Shimosato, Chief of the Pathology Division of the National Cancer Center Research Institute, Tokyo, Dr. Si-Chun Ming, Professor of the Department of Pathology, Temple University, Philadelphia, Pennsylvania, and Dr. C. Rubio, Associate Professor of the Department of Pathology, Karolinska Institute, Stockholm, for their helpful suggestions and reading of the manuscript. We thank Miss M. Yamamoto, Chief of Technicians in the Clinical Laboratory Division, and Mr. K. Ohnuki for their skillful technical assistance. We are also obliged to the members of the gastrointestinal tract study group of the National Cancer Center Hospital.

This work was supported in part by Grants-in-Aid for Cancer Research from the Ministry of Education (grant no. 58010091).

REFERENCES

1. Morson, B. C. Carcinoma arising from areas of intestinal metaplasia in the gastric mucosa. *Br. J. Cancer* 9 (1955):377–385.
2. Ming, S.-C., Goldman, H., and Freiman, D. G. Intestinal metaplasia and histogenesis of carcinoma in human stomach. *Cancer* 20 (1967):1418–1429.
3. Nakamura, K., Sugano, H., Takagi, K., and Kumakura, K. Histogenesis of carcinoma of the stomach with special reference to 50 primary microcarcinomas. Light- and electron-microscopic, and statistical studies. *Jpn. J. Cancer Clin.* 15 (1967):627–647.
4. Japanese Research Society for Gastric Cancer. The general rules for the gastric cancer study in surgery and pathology. *Jpn. J. Surg.* 6 (1976):69–78.
5. Bross, I. D. J. How to use ridit analysis. *Biometrics* 14 (1958):18–88.
6. Matsukura, N., Kawachi, T., Sugimura, T., Ohnuki, T., Higo, M., Itabashi, M., Hirota, T., and Kitaoka, H. Variety of phenotypical expression of intestinal marker enzymes and mucin in human stomach intestinal metaplasia. *Acta Histochem. Cytochem.* 13 (1980):499–507.
7. Hirota, T., Itabashi, M., Suzuki, K., and Yoshida, S. Clinico-pathologic study of minute and small early gastric cancer. Histogenesis of gastric cancer. *Pathol. Annu.* 15 (1980):1–9.
8. Ming, S.-C., and Goldman, H. Gastric polyps. A histogenetic classification and its relation to carcinoma. *Cancer* 18 (1965):721–726.

16 INTESTINAL METAPLASIA AND GASTRIC CARCINOMA

A. Gad

The long-postulated link between intestinal metaplasia and gastric carcinoma (1-3) has been supported by morphologic and epidemiologic studies. Gastric carcinoma has been consequently classified into intestinal, thought to arise in intestinal metaplasia, and diffuse (4). This classification has gained widespread acceptance and has been used in many epidemiologic studies, but several trials have been conducted to improve it (5, 6). The classification of gastric carcinoma on only a hypothetical histogenetic basis or according to the histological appearance of the tumor has proven to be of limited prognostic value.

At present, a universally accepted system of classification has not been developed, and the role of intestinal metaplasia in the pathogenesis of gastric carcinoma remains controversial. The evidence for an association between these two conditions is less firm than generally appreciated and deserves a critical review and reassessment. Light and electron microscopic studies as well as mucosubstance and enzyme histochemical investigations constitute the main bulk of the morphological evidence.

THE HISTOLOGICAL EVIDENCE

The histological evidence for a possible relationship between intestinal metaplasia and gastric carcinoma was founded on two sets of observations. Järvi and Laurén (1) noted the presence of a striated border on the surface of metaplastic and carcinoma cells. Morson (2) found that the incidence of intestinal metaplasia was higher in stomachs containing carcinomas than in those bearing ulcers, and that some tumors occurred in metaplastic areas (3).

The finding that carcinoma cells have features in common with intestinal metaplasia does not necessarily prove that they develop from benign metaplastic cells. Carcinomas may acquire intestinal or other characteristics during malignant transformation just as normal gastric epithelium may undergo metaplasia after exposure to injurious agents (7). In support of this, Paneth cells, not normally seen in gastric mucosa, were demonstrated in diffuse carcinomas, and glandular structures with brush border were often combined with individually infiltrating diffuse cells (8).

Intestinal metaplasia is so common that for practical purposes it cannot be regarded as a premalignant lesion. It was found in about 20 percent of a sample representing a large Finnish population. Its prevalence increases significantly with age, so that the expected frequency in Finnish people older than 60 years is about 40 percent (9). This stimulated attempts to delineate subtypes of intestinal metaplasia that could be more convincingly related histogenetically to carcinoma of the stomach. Incomplete intestinal metaplasia exhibiting features of both intestinal and gastric epithelium was described by Ming et al. (10) in 1967.

THE HISTOCHEMICAL EVIDENCE

Intestinal metaplasia, usually thought to resemble small intestine histologically and histochemically, was first divided into two types from a histochemical viewpoint—small intestinal and colonic (11). The colonic type was found to secrete O-acetylated sialomucins and to be associated with intestinal-type carcinoma. Jass and Filipe (12) and Jass (13) described a variant of intestinal metaplasia resembling the incomplete type of Ming and his collaborators (10) that secreted sulfomucin like colonic mucosa. The characteristics of the two main types of intestinal metaplasia are summarized in Table 16-1.

Later, Jass and Filipe (14) further divided incomplete metaplasia into sulfomucin-secreting subtype IIB and subtype IIA, producing a

Table 16-1.   Summary of the Characteristics of the
Two Main Types of Intestinal Metaplasia[a]

	Small Intestinal Type (Complete, Type I, or A)	Large Intestinal Type (Incomplete, Type II, or B)
Epithelium and crypts	Regular with occasional villi	Disturbed
Goblet cells	Frequent	Few
Endocrine and Paneth cells	Present	Absent
Brush border	Present and well formed	Absent
Mucosubstances	Neutral and sialomucins with traces of sulfomucins in goblet cells only	Sulfomucins in goblet and columnar cells
Enzymes	Small intestinal	Large intestinal
Distribution in the stomach	Major type	Minor type

[a]This is a summary of the data available in the literature.

mixture of neutral mucins and sialomucins with a trace of sulfomucin. The production of sulfomucin in intestinal metaplasia was interpreted by these authors as a sign of poor differentiation, which could be used as an indicator of a premalignant change related to the intestinal type of gastric carcinoma. This conclusion was founded on the incorrect belief that neutral mucin is characteristic of normal gastric mucosa and sialo- or sulfomucin of intestinal epithelium. Sulfomucin is one of the constituents of the bulk of mucosubstances of the normal stomach.

Sulfomucin was chemically detected in the gastric secretion from healthy young persons and from patients with histologically verified gastric cancer, peptic ulcers, and other gastric diseases (15). Histochemically it was demonstrated in the deep foveolar and mucous neck cells of the normal human stomach and in metaplastic cells in chronic gastritis (16, 17). All types of mucosubstances, neutral, sialo-, and sulfomucin, are secreted in relatively increased amounts by the surface epithelium and the gastric glands in the human fetus and neonate (17).

Sulfomucin is also produced under normal circumstances by the goblet cells of the distal ileum without this part being at increased risk for carcinoma compared with other parts of the small intestine that secrete sialomucin only (17). Sulfomucin was demonstrated in carcinoma of the small intestine irrespective of the part in which it arose (16). Even in the large intestine, the number of goblet cells secreting sulfomucins varies greatly from one part to the other and in neighboring crypts, with several segments being almost completely devoid of the substance. The normal left colonic and rectal mucosae secrete more sialomucin than sulfomucin (18).

In the lesion-free mucosa of a large number of stomachs resected for ulcer disease or carcinoma, the frequency of sulfomucin-secreting intestinal metaplasia was almost similar and did not vary significantly with the different types of carcinomas (17). No clear difference between the diffuse- and intestinal-type carcinomas has been noted regarding the secretion of sulfomucin. Well-differentiated and signet-ring-type carcinomas are known to produce sulfomucins (8, 18). It is therefore difficult to believe that the production of sulfomucin by gastric epithelial or metaplastic cells is a marker of premalignant change.

The present author has seen the various types and subtypes of intestinal metaplasia in the gastric mucosa of the same individual. In agreement with Sipponen and his collaborators (9, 19), it is suggested that these types are morphologically related and probably represent stages in a cycle of maturation and differentiation. In a recent study (19) the sensitivity and predictive value of colonic-type intestinal metaplasia as a risk factor for gastric carcinoma were found to be low.

Further indirect evidence supporting the view that intestinal metaplastic epithelium is of a precancerous nature stems from enzyme histochemical studies. Enzymes generally found only in the intestinal mucosa were detected both in gastric carcinoma and in intestinalized mucosa, and complete and incomplete variants have been also described in terms of patterns of enzyme synthesis (20). These findings may also be a manifestation of the process of malignant transformation, and have to be weighed against other results in this field that do not potentiate a relationship between intestinal metaplasia and gastric carcinoma. Several enzymes were found in gastric carcinomas that were not identified in mucous neck cells, pylorocardiac glands, or intestinal cells (21), and no appreciable difference in enzyme content was noted in differentiated and undifferentiated gastric carcinomas (22). To add to the complexity of the matter, the occurrence of intestinal-type gastric carcinoma was linked with a malignant transformation of intestinal metaplasia through a duodenal rather than a colonic pathway of differentiation (23, 24).

Tumor markers such as fetal sulfoglycoprotein antigen were demonstrated in intestinal and diffuse carcinomas (25), and intestinal mucosa-specific glycoprotein antigen was seen in diffuse carcinoma (26). Furthermore, placental alkaline phosphatase was found in intestinal metaplasia and gastric carcinoma as well as in hyperplastic states such as metaplastic polyps of the colon. This would point more to an association with any high cell turnover state, analogous to the production of high levels of carcinoembryonic antigen in inflammatory bowel disease (27), and not to a malignant potential.

THE ULTRASTRUCTURAL EVIDENCE

Ultrastructural similarity between intestinal-type carcinoma and metaplastic epithelium has been reported by many authors (10, 28, 29). Tall, well-developed microvilli forming the brush border on the apical cell surface are the common feature in intestinal metaplasia and gastric carcinoma, particularly the intestinal type. Two explanations for this resemblance are thought possible: Metaplastic changes may occur in the cells of the carcinomatous tissue, or the tumor may develop from intestinal metaplasia. There is a large body of evidence in disagreement with the latter.

The epithelium of complete metaplasia has been seen ultrastructurally to be identical to the intestinal epithelium, whereas that of the incomplete metaplasia possessed properties of both the gastric and intestinal epithelium (30). Most intestinal metaplasias consist of both types, and the incomplete variant finally develops into the complete one (31).

Both diffuse- and intestinal-type carcinomas were found to exhibit similar ultrastructural features. Intracellular cysts lined by microvilli were found in both types of carcinoma, and intestinal-like carcinoma without a brush border was described (8). Teglbjaerg (32) also reported a case of well-differentiated adenocarcinoma that originated in gastric epithelium. Ultrastructurally, the tumor cells were identical to the normal cells of the pyloric glands or the surface epithelium. However, microvilli normally occur in the cells of the pyloric glands (33), mucous neck cells, and foveolar epithelium (8).

Signet-ring cells have been ultrastructurally classified into types A, B, and C, and, especially those of type B, resemble the mucous neck and pyloric gland cells (34). Similar findings were reported earlier by Sasano et al. (35) who nevertheless concluded that most signet-ring cells were of the goblet cell type, a conclusion recently supported by two other studies (8, 29).

THE EXPERIMENTAL EVIDENCE

Intestinal metaplasia was induced in the pyloric glands of Wistar rats by local X-irradiation without being accompanied with or followed by the development of carcinoma (7). It was also found that the addition of mucosubstances to powerful carcinogenic agents diminishes the incidence of gastric carcinoma in experimental models of rodents and dogs preoperated with gastrojejunostomy (36, 37).

These interesting results indicate that metaplastic changes may represent a nonspecific response to various injurious agents, including carcinogens, and that mucosubstances protect the mucosa from the carcinogenic effect. It has been suggested earlier that the appearance of intestinal metaplastic cells in gastric mucosa may be a trial on the part of the stomach to increase its defenses by mobilizing new cells capable of secreting large amounts of mucosubstances in an altered milieu (17).

THE EPIDEMIOLOGICAL EVIDENCE

It has been claimed that the classification of gastric carcinoma into intestinal and diffuse types has proved useful in epidemiologic studies. The intestinal type differs from the diffuse in affecting an older age group, being more common among males, and having a better prognosis (4). It also dominates in countries with an especially high incidence of gastric carcinoma and in most of the excess incidence and mortality in subpopulations of migrants (38–42). It has also been reported (43) that when the gastric cancer risk is reduced in a population, it is the intestinal type of tumor that accounts for most of the reduction if the pylorus alone is taken into consideration. The reduction is slight and statistically insignificant if the tumors of the entire gastric epithelium are analyzed.

Recent studies from the United States, Japan, New Zealand, and Nigeria do not agree with these findings. Kubo (44–46) found similar proportions of the two types of cancer in high- and low-risk populations in the United States, Japan, and New Zealand. He also reported that age- and sex-specific proportions of diffuse gastric carcinoma do not vary with the overall gastric cancer incidence rates with time or place. An investigation in northern Nigeria, where gastric cancer is uncommon, revealed that intestinal-type carcinoma predominated in all age groups and in both sexes (47). It should be pointed out here that it is difficult to reconcile the high mortality rates owing to gastric carcinoma in high-risk areas in which intestinal-type carcinoma, said to have a better prognosis than the diffuse type, predominates.

These conflicting results are not easily explained, but innumerable sources of error and several methodological questions are involved. Epidemiologic studies were often based on autopsies, and one can imagine the enormous difficulties encountered in estimating the frequency of intestinal metaplasia and in typing cancers in such material. One of the most serious problems is the question of sampling and the amount of gastric mucosa examined, as it is well recognized that the distribution of intestinal metaplasia varies considerably from one part of the stomach to the other. Evaluation of unrepresentative material results in misleading judgments. Likewise, selection criteria for biopsy, surgery, and autopsy vary in different places to an extent that makes biased and uncomparable conclusions unavoidable when studying the incidence of gastric carcinoma. In interpreting results of studies conducted on migrants, it has to be remembered that, for various reasons, they may not be representative of the original population from which they derived.

Assuming that a representative sample is made available, one more obstacle remains to be overcome. This is related to the availability of a simple, meaningful, and reproducible classification system that makes uniform results from different parts of the world possible.

CLASSIFICATION OF GASTRIC CARCINOMA

Gastric carcinoma exhibits a wide variety of growth patterns and a great variability in the degree of differentiation even in different parts of the same tumor. Yet it is customary to describe a growth according to the predominating architecture without taking into consideration that certain types may carry a bad prognosis even when they constitute a minority of the cancer cell population. This is one of the shortcomings of most of the current classifications, which, perhaps for the sake of simplicity, lump gastric carcinoma into intestinal and diffuse (4), pylorocardiac, mucus cell, and intestinal (6), or expanding and infiltrative (5).

The identification of subgroups of gastric carcinoma may be useful in assessing the course and outcome of the disease as exemplified by the characterization and isolation of a group of neuroendocrine tumors. Similarly, it may be of prognostic value to consider such special types of tumors as carcinoma with lymphoid stroma and mucinous and signet-ring carcinomas as separate morphologic and prognostic entities. Mixed carcinomas should be also listed separately, and special attention should be paid to the various types present irrespective of whether they constitute minor or major elements. The classification put forward by the World Health Organization (48) divides gastric carcinoma into papillary, tubular, mucinous, and signet-ring types, but the tumor is named after the predominant type.

Other major prognostic factors include the spread of cancer through the wall of the stomach and the presence or absence of lymph node or distant metastases. Grundmann and Schlake (49) proposed a classification with emphasis on the maximum depth of invasion in the stomach wall and the vertical thickness of the tumor together with its histologic type and the predominant direction of spread. The value of staging gastric carcinoma in assessing survival has been statistically confirmed (50). In a series of gastric cancers reported from Japan (51), the 5-year survival rate of cancers limited to the mucosa or submucosa irrespective of lymph node metastasis averaged 95.5 percent. In another study (52) the 5-year survival rate was 50 percent when the tumor was confined to the submucosa, but fell to 20 percent when the muscle coat was penetrated.

Lymph node involvement in general is associated with a poor prognosis, the 5-year survival rate being 40.5 and 11.8 percent for node-negative and -positive patients, respectively (53). However, patients with metastases in a few lymph nodes have a better prognosis than those with metastases in many.

If the classification is to be meaningful, full clinical information and detailed examination of the resection specimens are necessary. The following data should be made available: the exact site of the tumor—whether cardiac, fundic, or pyloric; the depth of infiltration—mucosal, submucosal, in the muscle wall, or through it with extension in the surrounding adipose tissue; blood or lymph vessel permeation; and lymph node or distant metastases. The number of lymph nodes involved, their proximity to the site of the tumor, and the presence or absence of periglandular infiltration should be discussed.

The histological classification of gastric carcinoma shown in Table 16-2 has been used by this author for the last few years, and its prognostic value has been confirmed in a retrospective study using a large number of cases (to be published elsewhere). Pathologists are familiar with the diagnostic criteria of all tumor types included in this classification, as none of them is unique for gastric carcinoma. It should be a great advantage to use a unifying system of histological typing and grading applicable to adenocarcinoma irrespective of the organ or site of origin. Classifying signet-ring carcinomas in a special group and separating them from poorly differentiated adenocarcinomas is meaningful, as they disseminate more aggressively and carry a worse prognosis. The presence of signet-ring cells in a mixed carcinoma even as a minority cell population may lead to the same bad prognosis of a pure signet-ring carcinoma. The mixed tumors should therefore be looked upon as a heterogeneous group that may have a

Table 16-2. A Proposed Histological Classification of
Adenocarcinoma of the Stomach

Adenocarcinoma (not otherwise specified): Well differentiated; moderately differentiated; poorly differentiated
Signet-ring-type carcinoma
Mucinous carcinoma
Mixed carcinoma (any combination of the above-mentioned types; major and minor cell types noted)
Carcinoma with lymphoid stroma

prognosis equal to that of the most aggressive component. Terms such as "superficial" or "early" carcinoma are not used in this classification.

CONCLUSION

There is no convincing evidence to support the hypothesis that intestinal metaplasia is a premalignant lesion from which an intestinal-type adenocarcinoma of the stomach may arise. The classification of gastric carcinoma into intestinal and diffuse as well as other current classifications following a similar line are inadequate both histogenetically and prognostically.

To be of maximum benefit, a histological classification should be of value in the assessment of prognosis. A system found to fulfill this requirement is proposed, and the need for standardization of methods and criteria is emphasized. Histological classification and staging of gastric carcinoma are essential if valid comparisons of epidemiological or therapeutic results are to be made.

ACKNOWLEDGMENT

The assistance of the technical and secretarial staff of the Department of Clinical Pathology and Cytology, Falun Hospital, Falun, Sweden, in the preparation of this chapter is greatly appreciated.

REFERENCES

1. Järvi, O., and Laurén, P. On the role of heterotopias of the intestinal epithelium in the pathogenesis of gastric cancer. *Acta Pathol. Microbiol. Scand.* 29 (1951):26–43.

2. Morson, B. C. Intestinal metaplasia of the gastric mucosa. *Br. J. Cancer* 9 (1955):365–376.

3. Morson, B. C. Carcinoma arising from areas of intestinal metaplasia in the gastric mucosa. *Br. J. Cancer* 9 (1955):377–385.

4. Laurén, P. The two histological main types of gastric carcinoma: Diffuse and so-called intestinal type carcinoma. An attempt at a histoclinical classification. *Acta Pathol. Microbiol. Scand.* 64 (1965):31–49.

5. Ming, S.-C. Gastric carcinoma. A pathobiological classification. *Cancer* 30 (1977):2475–2485.

6. Mulligan, R. M. Histogenesis and biological behavior of gastric carcinoma. *Pathol. Annu.* 7 (1972):349–415.

7. Watanabe, H. Experimentally induced intestinal metaplasia in Eistar rats by X-ray irradiation. *Gastroenterology* 75 (1978):796–799.

8. Järvi, O., Nevalainen, T., Ekefors, T., and Kulatunga, A. The classification and histogenesis of gastric cancer. In *Proceedings of the XI International Cancer Congress Series. Tumors of Specific Sites, Vol. 354*, pp 228–234. Amsterdam: Excerpta Medica, 1975.

9. Sipponen, P., Seppälä, K., Varis, K., Hjelt, L., Ihamäki, T., Kekki, M., and Siurala, M. Intestinal metaplasia with colonic-type sulphomucins in the gastric mucosa; its association with gastric carcinoma. *Acta Pathol. Microbiol. Scand. (A)* 88 (1980):217–224.

10. Ming, S. -C., Goldman, H., and Freidman, D. G. Intestinal metaplasia and histogenesis of carcinoma in human stomach: Light and electron microscopic study. *Cancer* 20 (1967):1418–1429.

11. Teglbjaerg, P., and Nielsen, H. O. "Small intestinal type" and "colonic type" intestinal metaplasia of the human stomach, and their relationship to the histogenetic types of gastric adenocarcinoma. *Acta Pathol. Microbiol. Scand. (A)* 86 (1978):351–355.

12. Jass, J. R., and Filipe, M. I. Variants of intestinal metaplasia associated with gastric carcinoma. A histochemical study. *Histopathology* 3 (1979):191–199.

13. Jass, J. R. Role of intestinal metaplasia in the histogenesis of gastric carcinoma. *J. Clin. Pathol.* 33 (1980):801–809.

14. Jass, J. R., and Filipe, M. I. The mucin profiles of normal gastric mucosa, intestinal metaplasia and its variants and gastric carcinoma. *Histochem. J.* 13 (1981):931–939.

15. Häkkinen, I., and Viikarie, S. Occurrence of fetal sulphoglycoprotein antigen in the gastric juice of patients with gastric diseases. *Ann. Surg.* 169 (1969): 277–281.

16. Gad, A. Mucin histochemistry and questions in gastroenterology. *Scand. J. Gastroenterol.* 14, Suppl. 54 (1979):94–98.

17. Gad, A. Pathophysiology of gastrointestinal mucins. *Adv. Physiol. Sci.* 29 (1981):161–184.

18. Gad, A. A histochemical study of human alimentary tract mucosubstances in health and disease. I. Normal and tumors. *Br. J. Cancer* 23 (1969):52–63.

19. Sipponen, P. Intestinal metaplasia and gastric carcinoma. *Ann. Clin. Res.* 13 (1981):139–143.

20. Kawachi, T., Kurisu, M., Numanyu, N., Sasajima, K., Sano, T., and Sugimura, T. Precancerous changes in the stomach. *Cancer Res.* 36 (1976):2673–2677.

21. Planteydt, H. T., and Willighagen, R. G. J. Enzyme histochemistry of the human stomach with special reference to intestinal metaplasia. *J. Pathol. Bacteriol.* 80 (1960):713–722.

22. Stemmermann, G. N., and Hayashi, T. Intestinal metaplasia of the gastric mucosa. A gross and microscopic study of its distribution in various disease states. *J. Natl. Cancer Inst.* 41 (1968):627–634.
23. Bara, J., Hamelin, L., Martin, E., and Burtin, P. Intestinal M3 antigen, a marker for the intestinal type differentiation of gastric carcinomas. *Int. J. Cancer* 28 (1981):711–719.
24. Nardelli, J., Bara, J., Rosa, B., and Burtin, P. Intestinal metaplasia and carcinomas of the human stomach: An immunohistochemical study. *J. Histochem. Cytochem.* 31 (1983):366–375.
25. Häkkinen, I., Järvi, O., and Grönroos, J. Sulphoglycoprotein antigens in the human alimentary canal and gastric cancer. An immunological study. *Int. J. Cancer* 3 (1968):572–581.
26. Kawasaki, H., Imasato, K., Kimoto, E., Akiyama, K., and Takeuchi, M. Immunohistological studies on intestinal mucosa-specific glycoprotein in gastric carcinoma. *Gann* 63 (1972):231–237.
27. Skinner, J. M., and Whitehead, R. Carcinoplacental alkaline phosphatase in malignant and premalignant conditions of the human digestive tract. *Virchows Arch. (Pathol. Anat.)* 394 (1981):109–118.
28. Goldman, H., and Ming, S. -C. Fine structure of intestinal metaplasia and adenocarcinoma of the human stomach. *Lab. Invest.* 18 (1968):203–210.
29. Nevalainen, T. J., and Järvi, O. H. Ultrastructure of intestinal and diffuse type gastric carcinoma. *J. Pathol.* 122 (1977):129–136.
30. Iida, F., Murata, F., and Nagata, T. Histochemical studies of mucosubstances in metaplastic epithelium of the stomach, with special reference to the development of intestinal metaplasia. *Histochemistry* 56 (1978):229–237.
31. Iida, F., and Kusama, J. Gastric carcinoma and intestinal metaplasia. Significance of types of intestinal metaplasia upon development of gastric carcinoma. *Cancer* 50 (1982):2854–2858.
32. Teglbjaerg, P. S. Highly differentiated gastric adenocarcinoma originating from the normal, non-metaplastic gastric epithelium. An ultrastructural study of a case. *Acta Pathol. Microbiol. Scand. (A)* 86 (1978):87–89.
33. Rubin, W., Ross, L. L., Sleisenger, M. H., and Jeffries, G. H. The normal human gastric epithelia. A fine structural study. *Lab. Invest.* 19 (1968):598–626.
34. Yamashiro, K., Suzuki, H., and Nagay, T. Electron microscopic study of signet-ring cells in diffuse carcinoma of the human stomach. *Virchows Arch. (Pathol. Anat.)* 374 (1977):275–284.
35. Sasano, N., Nakamura, K., Arai, M., and Akazaki, K. Ultrastructural cell patterns in human gastric carcinoma compared with non-neoplastic gastric mucosa. Histogenetic analysis of carcinoma by mucin histochemistry. *J. Natl. Cancer Inst.* 43 (1969):783–802.
36. Dahm, K., and Werner, B. Susceptibility of the resected stomach to experimental carcinogenesis. *Z. Tschr. Krebsforsch.* 85 (1976):219–229.
37. Tatematsu, M., Takahashi, M., Hananouchi, M., Shirai, T., Hirose, M., Fukushirora, S., and Ito, N. Protective effect of mucin in experimental gastric cancer induced by N-methyl-N'-nitro-N-nitrosoguanidine plus sodium chloride in rats. *Gann* 67 (1976):223–229.
38. Correa, P., Cuello, E., and Duque, E. Carcinoma and intestinal metaplasia of the stomach in Colombian migrants. *J. Natl. Cancer Inst.* 44 (1970):297–306.
39. Correa, P., Sasano, N., Stemmermann, G. N., and Haenszel, W. Pathology of gastric carcinoma in Japanese populations: Comparison between Miyagi prefecture, Japan and Hawaii. *J. Natl. Cancer Inst.* 51 (1973):1449–1459.

40. Munoz, N. and Connelly, R. Time trends of intestinal and diffuse types of gastric cancer in the United States. *Int. J. Cancer* 8 (1971):158–164.
41. Munoz, N., and Asvall, J. Time trends in intestinal and diffuse types of gastric cancer in Norway. *Int. J. Cancer* 8 (1971):144–157.
42. Munoz, N., Correa, P., Cuello, C., and Duque, E. Histologic types of gastric carcinoma in high and low risk areas. *Int. J. Cancer* 3 (1968):809–818.
43. Kato, Y., Kiagawa, T., Nakamura, K., and Sugano, H. Changes in the types of gastric carcinoma in Japan. *Cancer* 48 (1981):2084–2087.
44. Kubo, T. Gastric carcinoma in New Zealand: Some epidemiologic-pathologic aspects. *Cancer* 31 (1973):1498–1507.
45. Kubo, T. Geographical pathology of gastric carcinoma. *Acta Pathol. Jpn.* 24 (1974):465–479.
46. Kubo, T. Histologic appearance of gastric carcinoma in high and low mortality countries: Comparison between Kyushu, Japan and Minnesota, USA. *Cancer* 28 (1971):726–734.
47. Mabogunje, O. A., Subbuswamy, S. G., and Lawrie, J. H. The two histological types of gastric carcinoma in northern Nigeria. *Gut* 19 (1978):425–429.
48. WHO. Histological typing of gastric and oesophageal tumours. International histological classification of tumours, No. 18. Geneva: World Health Organization, 1977.
49. Grundmann, E., and Schlake, W. Histological classification of gastric cancer from initial to advanced stages. *Pathol. Res. Pract.* 173 (1982):260–274.
50. Kennedy, B. J. TNM classification for stomach cancer. *Cancer* 26 (1970):971–983.
51. Kidokoro, T. Frequency of resection, metastasis and five-year survival rate of early gastric carcinoma in a surgical clinic. *Gann Monogr. Cancer Res.* 11 (1971):45–49.
52. Paile, A. Morphology and prognosis of carcinoma of the stomach. *Ann. Chir. Gynaecol. Fenn.* 60, Suppl. 175 (1977):1–56.
53. Hawley, P. R., Westerholm, P., and Morson, B. C. Pathology and prognosis of carcinoma of the stomach. *Brit. J. Surg.* 57 (1970):877–883.

17 THE POSSIBLE MODE OF APPEARANCE OF FETAL ANTIGEN EXPRESSIONS IN MUCOUS GASTRIC GLYCOPROTEINS

I. P. T. Häkkinen and O. H. Järvi

The mucus film on the surface of the gastric mucosa consists of glycoprotein macromolecules possessing a tendency to aggregate on the "visible" mucus. The glycoproteins themselves are the synthesis product of the superficial mucous cells, and can also be found in the gastric juice as dissolved macromolecules. In the cell membranes of the secreting cells, the same glycoprotein structures can be shown to be tightly bound. Earlier investigators took great pains in their attempts to elucidate the essence of "visible" and invisible mucus, without finding any final sense. However, recent investigations of the identity of the antigenic structures in glycoproteins in these three locations have clarified the picture. It may be significant that one part of the molecules is an aggregate of the physicochemical surface film, but it is certainly important that some macromolecules are present in the free gastric juice as dissolved single units—they are probably not degradation products, otherwise more polydispersity would be observed under normal conditions.

The antigenic structure of gastric mucous glycoproteins contains known blood group antigens (1), but the same molecules also contain oncogenetically organ-specific antigens (2, 3). The recent observation of changes in these organ-specific antigens under various pathological conditions lends them a special interest. Gastric mucous glycoproteins during the fetal period differ antigenically from the adult forms, although, immunohistologically, even adult structures are present in the fetal mucous cradle. Although normally absent from the adult mucous cells, fetal glycoprotein structures can reappear in transformation such as during carcinogenesis. This is well in accordance with the general concept of cell transformation. In humans this information can be collected only from a maze of single observations. Quite recently, however, an experimental model effected by the known carcinogen N-methyl-N'-nitro-N-nitrosoguanidine has been presented (4) that throws light on the course of the events during carcinogenesis.

FETAL SIALOGLYCOPROTEIN ANTIGEN OF HUMAN GASTRIC JUICE

Soluble glycoproteins of the gastric juice are good starting materials for purification and characterization, and two series of studies concerning their properties have been published recently (5, 6). Immunohistologically, the neutral glycoproteins seem to localize mainly in the deep parts of the gastric glands (7, 8). Their characterization still needs complete studies, but interest has been paid primarily to the acid glycoproteins of the superficial gastric mucosa. In the case of a young healthy adult, the physicochemical and immunochemical structures of the acid gastric glycoproteins are rather homogeneous. They are characterized by uniformly large molecular size as seen from disc electrophoresis (5) and the antigen we call N_O antigen prevailing as the organ-specific marker (2), together with the known ABO blood group antigens.

With advancing age, however, morphological changes quite frequently appear in the gastric mucosa of humans. Whatever the cause, the fact is that the stomach is markedly affected by both outer and inner agents. Changes are also observable in the antigenic structure of acid glycoproteins of the gastric juice.

Table 17-1. The Chemical Composition
and Molecular Weight of Fetal
Sialoglycoprotein Antigen of Gastric Juice

Compounds	%
Galactose	13.5
Fucose	7.4
Sialic acid	5.4
Sulfate	Trace
Glucosamine	24.5
Galactosamine	16.9
Amino acids	32.3
Aspartic acid	2.1
Threonine	5.6
Serine	3.2
Glutamic acid	2.9
Proline	2.6
Glycine	1.6
Alanine	1.6
Cystine	0.4
Valine	1.6
Isoleucine	1.7
Leucine	1.6
Tyrosine	0.4
Phenylalanine	0.6
Lysine	1.2
Histidine	0.5
Arginine	1.2
Cysteine + cystine	1.9
Tryptophan	0.8
Molecular weight,	160,000 daltons.

Using immunochemical methods it has been possible to find a macromolecule among the acid gastric glycoproteins that is characterized by the relationship it has with both the fetal period and the appearance of cancer. The compound is called fetal sialoglycoprotein antigen (FSA) (9; Table 17-1). The occurrence of this marker in the gastric juice of Finnish populations has been studied using a qualitative microimmunodiffusion method (10). Industrial workers in the age range of 40 to 64 years showed a rate of 3.5 percent for FSA secretion; among an unselected rural population in the age range of 40 to 70 years, the figure was 8.5 percent. Gastroscopy performed on the FSA secretors yielded a number of silent and mostly operable gastric cancers, the amount corresponding to the incidence rate in the area that was investigated. About 50 percent of the cancer cases were early can-

Table 17-2. Clinical Findings (Gastroscopy)
in 3,508 Fetal Sialoglycoprotein
Antigen-Positive Subjects from 39,706
Rural People Aged 40 to 70 Years

Gastroscopy Finding and Histological Diagnosis	No. of Cases
Gastric cancer	35
Gastric carcinoid	1
Tubular adenoma	10
Atrophic gastritis	346
Superficial gastritis	
Verified by biopsy	250
No biopsy	614
Erosive gastritis/gastric erosion	43
Peptic ulcer	45
Polyp(s)	153

cers not spread beyond the submucosa (11). Among the clinical findings there was also a wide variation of benign pathological conditions,
indicating the need for a follow-up investigation for the possibility of
developing malignancy (12; Table 17-2).

EXPERIMENTAL CHEMICAL CARCINOGENESIS AND FETAL EXPRESSIONS

Employing a previously described purification technique using ce-
tylpyridinium chloride precipitation of the polyanionic compounds,
it was possible to separate and purify characteristic glycoprotein frac-
tions from extracts of fetal canine intestinal mucosa. The immuniza-
tion of rabbits resulted in antisera apparently directed against these
glycoprotein structures (4). Immunohistologically, these antisera recognized the structures localized in the cell membranes and adjacent
mucus of the superficial fetal gastric mucous cells. In adult dogs the
corresponding structures could not be recognized. On the other
hand, using glycoproteins from gastric juice of healthy adult dogs as
the immunogen, antisera were raised that recognized these adult
structures (Figures 17-1 and 17-2). One large dose of N-methyl-N'-ni-
tro-N-nitrosoguanidine (600 milligrams) was given via an oral tube to
four adult beagle dogs. Its effect was followed by regular sampling of
gastric juice specimens and taking biopsies on gastroscopy under an-
esthesia during a total follow-up time of 15.5 months. The dogs were
maintained for 36 months, after which the stomachs at autopsy were

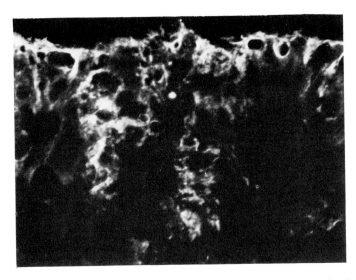

Figure 17-1.   Immunohistological localization of specific rabbit antibodies raised against glycoproteins of fetal canine alimentary mucosa, in the gastric mucosa of a fetal dog. Immunofluorescence of an antirabbit sheep fluorescein conjugate. × 63.

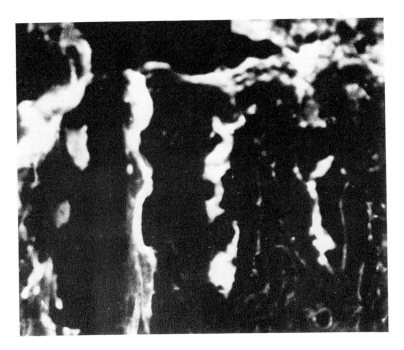

Figure 17-2.   Gastric mucosa of an adult healthy dog. Immunohistological localization of specific rabbit antibodies raised against glycoproteins of the gastric juice of a healthy adult dog. × 75.

investigated both macroscopically and histologically. No signs of existing malignancy or gastritis could be verified. However, immunodiffusion analysis of the glycoproteins present in the gastric juice specimens using antisera prepared against fetal structures revealed a gradually changing picture in each dog. Over a period of time, new fetal structures cross-reacting with the previous components appeared in the gastric glycoproteins of the dogs. The change continued throughout the observation period of 15.5 months.

When immunohistological methods were used, spots of positive fetal staining were observed both in the biopsies and in the final autopsy specimens. These stains were localized in the superficial epithelial cells, and in some sections positive staining was even found in the upper part of the glands extending to the neck cell area of the generating cells (Figure 17-3). As a control to check that the observed changes were not caused by unspecific irritation, the specimens were tested with earlier prepared antisera to glycoproteins of canine gastric juice after aspirin feeding of the dog (13). No recognition of fetal structures was observed.

In search of a rationale for the above observations, we have to think about the effect of *N*-methyl-*N'*-nitro-*N*-nitrosoguanidine in our experiment. We know that the compound reacts immediately with proteins and nucleoproteins, thus losing its chance for further similar

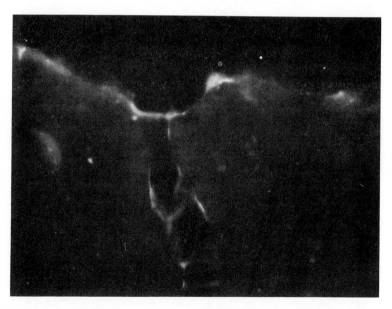

Figure 17-3.   Gastric mucosa of an adult dog 11.5 months after administration of a single dose of *N*-methyl-*N'*-nitro-*N*-nitrosoguanidine. The specific antibodies are seen as positive fluorescent spots. Same reagents used as in Figure 17-1. × 63.

reaction. The glycoproteins of the gastric mucous surface form a first barrier where a part of the applied substance is apparently halted. If the dose is large enough, saturation will be reached in the mucosa, and before long the important neck cell area with its generating cell population is exposed. Once transformed, the generating mother cells on dividing pass on their inheritance—in this case, the expression of fetal glycoproteins. As a function of time, these daughter cells increase in number and occupy the upper mouth of the gastric glands and the surrounding area in accordance with the general concept of epithelial cell renewal described recently by Fujita and Wattori (14). The observation of a stepwise increase of fetal structures among the gastric glycoproteins during a prolonged period of time could find its explanation in this way—by an increase in the amount of transformed daughter cells bearing these fetal properties. It is also possible that from one cell generation to another, the existing transformation takes on new characters although additional carcinogen is no longer available.

In our experiment none of the dogs developed cancer or chronic gastritis. Signs of acute inflammation of the gastric mucosa were ob-

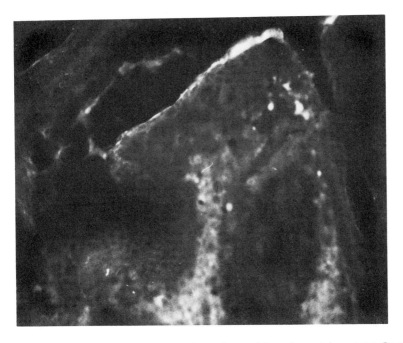

Figure 17-4. Human gastric mucosa of a patient with early gastric cancer. Section outside cancerous invasion. Immunohistological localization of specific rabbit antifetal sialoglycoprotein antigen antibodies seen as positive fluorescent spots in the mucosal surface. × 63.

served in the beginning of the experiment, but disappeared in later specimens. Apparently, N-methyl-N'-nitro-N-nitrosoguanidine has an unspecific irritative effect in addition to its specific mutagenic/carcinogenic effect. For development of a carcinoma in a dog, daily administration over a prolonged period of 1 to 1.5 years is necessary. The question of if this is necessary for the effect of mutagenity/carcinogenity then arises. The other unspecific effect leading to chronic irritation and gastritis may be as important. In this case the concept of Fujita and Wattori (14) concerning the development of gastric cancer could involve two components: the mutagen and the splitting of the gastric architecture by chronic irritation.

Very recently, we studied a surgical specimen of a cancerous stomach resulting from our mass screening. The alteration was a very early, intramucosal, diffuse-type, carcinomatous infiltration, discernible only microscopically over an area of 3 by 1.5 centimeters. The immunohistological localization of FSA in the area outside the cancerous infiltration was very similar to that observed in our experiment with dogs (Figure 17-4).

REFERENCES

1. Buchanan, D. J. and Rapoport, S. A chemical study of the blood group-specific substances found in meconium. *J. Biol. Chem.* 192 (1951):251–260.
2. Häkkinen, I., and Virtanen, S. The appearance of blood group and organ-specific antigens in human gastric glycoproteins. *Int. Arch. Allergy Appl. Immunol.* 39 (1970):272–279.
3. Häkkinen, I. P. T. Gastric fetal sulphoglycoprotein antigen (FSA) and blood group antigens A and B. *Int. Arch. Allergy Appl. Immunol.* 47 (1974):380–387.
4. Häkkinen, I. P. T., Heinonen, R., Isberg, U., and Järvi, O. H. Canine gastric glycoprotein antigens in early carcinogenesis. *Cancer* (in press).
5. Häkkinen, I. An immunochemical method for detecting carcinomatous secretion from human gastric juice. *Scand. J. Gastroenterol.* 1 (1966):28–32.
6. Häkkinen, I. P. T. FSA—Foetal sulphoglycoprotein antigen associated with gastric cancer. *Transplant. Rev.* 20 (1974):61–76.
7. Häkkinen, I., Järvi, O., and Grönroos, J. Sulphoglycoprotein antigents in the human alimentary canal and gastric cancer. *Int. J. Cancer* 3 (1968):572–581.
8. Häkkinen, I., and Laitio, M. Epithelial glycoproteins of human gallbladder. Immunological characterization. *Arch. Pathol.* 90 (1970):137–142.
9. Häkkinen, I. The purification procedure for human gastric juice FSA and its chemical composition. *Clin. Exp. Immunol.* 42 (1980):57–62.
10. Häkkinen, I. P. T. Foetal sulphoglycoprotein antigen (FSA) as a possible precursor of alimentary canal cancers. *Scand. J. Gastroenterol.* 7 (1972):483–488.
11. Häkkinen, I. P. T., Heinonen, R., Inberg, M. V., Järvi, O. H., Vaajalahti, P., and Viikari, S. Clinicopathological study of gastric cancers and precancerous states detected by fetal sulfoglycoprotein antigen screening. *Cancer Res.* 40 (1980):4308–4312.

12. Häkkinen, I. Application of serum and gastric juice tumour markers to early diagnosis and screening of gastric cancer. In *Gastric Cancer*, edited by Fielding, J. W., pp 85–94. Oxford: Pergamon Press, 1981.

13. Häkkinen, I. P. T., Johansson, R., and Pantio, M. An immunological and histoimmunological study of gastric sulphoglycoproteins in healthy and aspirin-treated dogs. *Gut* 9 (1968):712–716.

14. Fujita, S., and Hattori, T. Cell proliferation, differentiation, and migration in the gastric mucosa: A study on the background of carcinogenesis. In *Pathophysiology of Carcinogenesis in Digestive Organs*, edited by Farber, E., Kawachi, T., Nagayo, T., Sugano, H., Sugimura, T., and Weisburger, J. H., pp 21–36. Tokyo: University of Tokyo Press, 1977.

V POLYPS

18 MALIGNANT POTENTIAL OF EPITHELIAL POLYPS OF THE STOMACH

S.-C. Ming

Gastric polyps have been considered precancerous for a long time. The reported incidence of malignant change in polyps varied greatly, however, until it was recognized that gastric polyps were heterogeneous and that their malignant potential was related to their histological composition. The first attempt to classify polyps histologically was made in 1945 when Rieniets and Broders (1) divided gastric polyps into two types: adenomas and papillary adenomas. Malignant change was common in the latter. In 1955 Morson (2) divided them into two types also. One type was composed of intestinal epithelium and the other gastric epithelium. Carcinoma was more common in the former type. In 1965 Ming and Goldman (3) classified them into a neoplastic type with high malignant potential and a nonneoplastic type with low malignant potential. The former was called adenomatous and the latter regenerative. At the same time they called attention to an increased incidence of coexisting but independent carcinoma in the polyp-containing stomach. There have been other classifications (4–7), using different terminology but with similar implications.

Table 18-1. Classifications of Gastric Polyps

Reference	Classification				
Elster (6)	Focal foveolar hyperplasia	Hyperplasiogenous polyp	Adenoma, high differentiation	Adenoma, moderate differentiation	Borderline lesion, protruded
Koch et al. (7)	Polypoid foveolar hyperplasia	Hyperplastic polyp	Hyperplastic adenomatous polyp	Villous polyp / Adenomatous villous polyp	—
Nakamura (5)	Type 2	Type 1	—	—	Type 3
Ming (8)	Hyperplastic (regenerative) polyp			Papillary (villous) adenoma	Flat adenoma

HISTOLOGIC CLASSIFICATIONS OF GASTRIC POLYPS

Some of the classifications of gastric polyps are compared in Table 18-1. Focal foveolar hyperplasia is a common nonspecific lesion, as pointed out by Elster (6). In the majority of cases, it is seen in nonpolypoid conditions. When it does form a polypoid lesion, it may be considered to be an early phase of hyperplastic polyp (8). The usual hyperplastic polyp is composed mostly of hyperplastic and often dilated foveolae. In the well-developed lesion, groups of pyloric glands are commonly found in the deep portion of the polyp. The latter type of lesion has been called adenoma or adenomatous (6, 7). The adenoma-like congregation of glands does not have the cellular characteristics of a truly neoplastic adenoma, however. Thus, the hyperplastic polyp has a wide range of component cells, all of which are histologically hyperplastic but otherwise normal.

The adenomas are composed of dysplastic glands with moderate differentiation. They often have a papillary or villous contour. A type of slightly elevated superficial tubular adenoma has been called a flat adenoma (8, 9). This lesion was initially called simply an atypical epithelium (10) or a borderline lesion (6, 10, 11) because the glands are lined by atypical cells, the benignity or malignancy of which is sometimes uncertain. Such a lesion has also been called IIa-like (11) or a IIa-subtype (12) lesion because it is reminiscent of Type IIa early carcinoma (10).

In addition to the hyperplastic (regenerative) polyp and adenoma, there are three other less common histological types of gastric polyps: hamartomatous, retention, and heterotopic (8). These five types are all epithelial polyps, meaning that they are composed pri-

marily of epithelial tissue. The inflammatory polyp is usually not included in this category, because it is made mainly of inflamed stromal
tissue. The glands in an inflammatory polyp are often dilated but usually not increased. Inflammatory polyps constituted 36 percent (130
cases) of 357 gastric polyps found among 13,200 gastroscopic examinations by Laxén et al. (13). Carcinoma was found in the stomach, outside the polyp, in three cases. There was no malignant change of the
inflammatory polyp itself. In contrast, malignant changes do occur in
epithelial polyps with varying frequency. Earlier accounts of these
changes have been reported (8). More recent information is presented
below.

HYPERPLASTIC POLYP

Hyperplastic polyp is the most common polyp in the stomach, comprising 75 to 90 percent of gastric polyps (8). The reported incidence
of malignant change within the polyp varies from 0 to 4 percent and
coexisting carcinoma outside the polyp from 8 to 28 percent. In the
more recent reports, hyperplastic polyp accounted for 86 to 97 percent of epithelial polyps (7, 13, 14) with different percentages of cases
in the subgroups. In Rösch's report (14) there were 248 hyperplasiogenic polyps and only 42 hyperplastic polyps. In the report by
Koch et al. (7), there were 763 cases of polypoid foveolar hyperplasia
with dysplasia I in 39, dysplasia II in 27, dysplasia III in 8, and associated cancer in 18. Among 21 cases of hyperplastic polyps, there was 1
case each with dysplasia I or II. Among 20 cases of hyperplastic adenomatous polyp, there were 2 cases each with dysplasia I or II. (See
Oehlert's grading system of dysplasia in Chapter 2). There was no example of malignant change in any of them. In the report by Laxén et
al. (13) there were 123 cases of hyperplastic polyp and 75 cases of
foveolar hyperplasia. There were two cases each in each group with
cancer in the polyp and five and four cases, respectively, of cancer
outside the polyp. The different usage of terms and the great variation
in numbers of cases in these reports indicate that these subtypes have
a common histological pattern and are related.

Carcinoma in the hyperplastic polyp was also reported by Nagayo (15) in 1 (0.6 percent) of 175 cases and by Yamagata and Hisamichi (16) in 5 (2.1 percent) of 236 operated cases. The latter authors also followed 974 patients: None developed cancer. The
incidence of malignancy in the total of 1,210 cases was 0.4 percent.

Kozuka et al. (17) divided gastric polyps into gastric and metaplastic types, presumably corresponding to the hyperplastic polyp and
adenoma. Carcinoma was found in 2 (0.08 percent) of 237 pure gas-

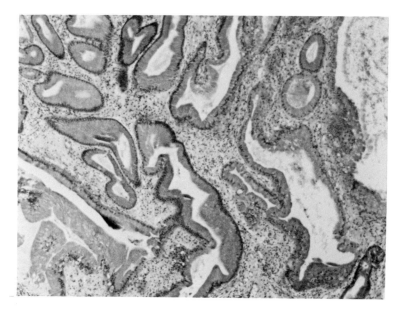

Figure 18-1.   Hyperplastic polyp. The tortuous foveolae are lined by mature mucous cells. H&E stain. × 80.

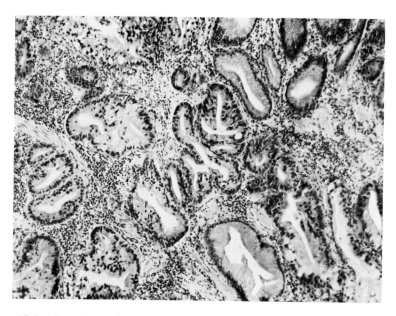

Figure 18-2.   Dysplastic glands and hyperplastic foveolae (**right**) in a hyperplastic polyp. H&E stain. × 80.

tric-type polyps, 14 (10.9 percent) of 128 gastric-type polyps with secondary metaplasia, and 32 (72.7 percent) of 44 metaplastic polyps.

Follow-up studies were done by Mizuno et al. (18) on 118 patients. Cancer developed in four cases: one in a hyperplastic polyp in
1.5 years, one in an adenoma in 2 years, and two in 2.1 and 3.5 years
without prior biopsy. The polyp increased in size in seven and decreased in size in four cases. Kawai et al. (19) found carcinoma in 1 of
75 polyps followed for 3 years but none in 38 cases followed for 6 to
15 years. Laxén et al. (13) followed 161 cases (including cases with
inflammatory polyps) for an average of 2.5 (up to 5) years. The number of polyps increased in 19 percent, decreased in 7 percent, and
disappeared in 14 percent.

In most reports the development of carcinoma in the polyp was
not illustrated. Remmele and Kolb (20) reported the finding of carcinoma in two of three hyperplastic polyps in a 71-year-old female.
The microphotographs showed both cancerous and hyperplastic
glands in the same lesion.

It is evident that hyperplastic polyps may undergo malignant
change, but the incidence is very low. There has been virtually no information about the transformation process itself. The hyperplastic
polyp is composed of mature and well-differentiated foveolar and
glandular cells (Figure 18-1). Such cells do not become malignant un-

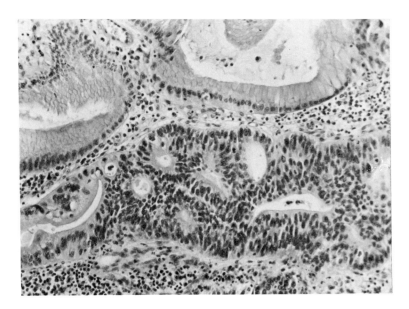

Figure 18-3.   Adenomatous tissue (**bottom**) and hyperplastic foveolae (**top**) in a hyperplastic polyp. H&E stain. × 240.

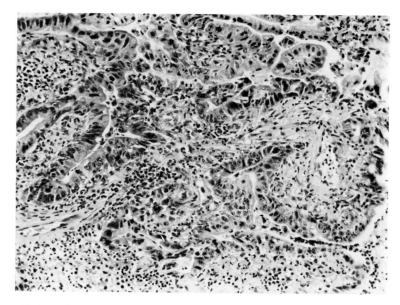

Figure 18-4.   Adenocarcinoma in the polyp shown in Figure 18-3. H&E stain. × 240.

der ordinary circumstances. There are at least two possibilities, however, by which the hyperplastic polyp may be converted to a precancerous lesion. One is the occurrence of dysplastic change (Figure 18-2) and the other is adenomatous change (Figures 18-3 and 18-4). Whether these changes are separate or variations of one process is at the present time difficult to determine because of inadequate materials. In view of these possibilities, the hyperplastic polyps may be subdivided into three types as listed in Table 18-2. The incidence of

Table 18-2. Subtypes of Hyperplastic Polyps
of the Stomach and Their
Variable Composition

Simple hyperplastic polyp
Polypoid foveolar hyperplasia
Foveolar + glandular hyperplasia
Foveolar + glandular + stromal hyperplasia
Dysplastic (adenomatous) hyperplastic polyp
Hyperplasia + dysplasia
Hyperplasia + adenoma
Malignant hyperplastic polyp
Hyperplasia + dysplasia + carcinoma
Hyperplasia + adenoma + carcinoma
Hyperplasia + carcinoma

the dysplastic type, according to Koch et al. (7), is about 5 percent (38 of 804 polyps had dysplasia II or III). The average incidence of malignancy in the reports cited above, excluding that of Kozuka et al. (17), is about 0.4 percent.

ADENOMA

Adenoma reportedly comprised about 10 to 25 percent of gastric polyps and malignant change occurred in 6 to 75 percent of them with an average of 41 percent (8). In the recent reports, adenoma was found in 2.7 to 12.8 percent of epithelial gastric polyps (7, 13, 14, 16) and was the seat of carcinoma in 10.4 percent of early gastric cancers (21). Types of adenoma varied. Gastric adenomas in Japan were mainly the flat type (16, 22) with malignant change within in 5 to 13 percent as in earlier reports. The metaplastic polyps reported by Kozuka et al. (17) were probably also flat adenomas, but malignancy was found in 32 (72.7 percent) of 44 metaplastic adenomas, a very high incidence. Koch et al. (7) had 18 cases of villous polyp and 8 cases of adenomatous villous polyp. One of the latter cases had an associated carcinoma. Carcinoma within the adenoma was not described.

It is interesting to note that the geographical differences for flat and papillary (villous) adenomas persist. The flat adenoma is a form of tubular adenoma (9). Its peculiar localization in the superficial region of gastric mucosa (Figures 18-5 and 18-6) distinguishes it from the larger polypoid adenomas that have a papillary or villous pattern (Figure 18-7). The histological appearance of a flat adenoma therefore resembles a dysplastic epithelium. That is the reason for its original

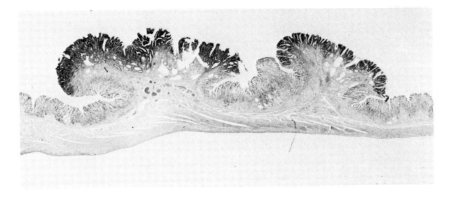

Figure 18-5.   Scanning view of two flat adenomas which are shown as dark tissue in the superficial portion of the gastric mucosa. H&E stain. × 7.

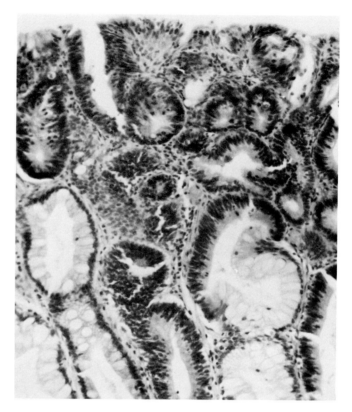

Figure 18-6. Flat adenoma. The adenomatous tissue occupies the superficial portion of the gastric mucosa. The mucosa below shows intestinal metaplasia. Abrupt transition from normal to adenomatous cells is seen in one gland. H&E stain. × 200.

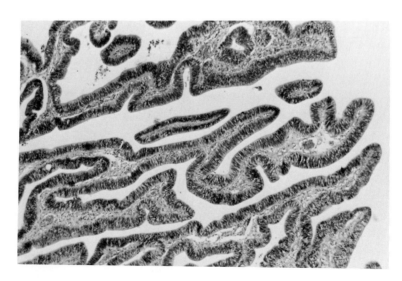

Figure 18-7. Papillovillous adenoma. Note the uniformity of the adenomatous cells. H&E stain. × 80.

Table 18-3. Differences between Flat Adenoma and
Dysplastic Epithelium of the Stomach

Characteristics	Flat Adenoma	Dysplastic Epithelium
Nature	Neoplasm	Not a neoplasm
Abnormal cells	Relatively uniform	Variable in abnormality
Junction with adjacent cell	Abrupt	Gradual and indistinct
Location	Superficial mucosa	Whole mucosa, more severe at bottom
Outline	Sharp	Indefinite
Regression	Not likely	Possible
Background mucosa	Incomplete metaplasia common	Atrophic gastritis common

name of "atypical epithelium" (10) and subsequent name of "border-line lesion" (6, 11). However, there are important differences between a flat adenoma and a dysplastic epithelium (Table 18-3). The flat adenoma, being a neoplasm, is sharply demarcated both grossly and microscopically with an abrupt border (Figure 18-6). The adenomatous cells are quite uniform, whereas the degree of abnormality is often variable in the dysplastic epithelium. The adenoma may change in size (22) but does not disappear. Regression is possible for the dysplastic epithelium (23). Malignant change occurs in both conditions: The incidence in adenoma is about 10 percent (16, 22). The incidence of malignancy in the dysplastic epithelium is unknown, but probably lower. The tendency of flat adenoma cells toward malignancy has been detected by electron microscopy by Riemann et al. (24). The flat adenoma is often surrounded by an incompletely metaplastic mucosa with only mild chronic inflammation, whereas dysplasia commonly occurs in chronic atrophic gastritis where the inflammation is often intense.

A detailed study of the flat adenoma is presented in Chapter 19.

HAMARTOMATOUS POLYP

The hamartomatous polyp is composed of an excessive amount of normally present tissue in a disorderly arrangement. Thus, the hamartomatous polyp of the stomach is made of gastric, not intestinal, tissue. Three types are recognized: Peutz-Jeghers, juvenile, and fundic gland. They are seen usually in hereditary diseases. Malignant change occurs rarely or not at all in these polyps.

The most likely candidate for malignant change is the Peutz-Jeghers polyp. Such instances have been reported in the stomach, but convincing evidence has not been presented (8). This situation applies to malignant transformation in the intestines as well. Recently, however, Cochet et al. (25) documented dysplastic and cancerous changes in Peutz-Jeghers polyps of the duodenum and stomach in a mother and her son. Both of them died of metastasizing cancers—duodenal in the mother and gastric in the son. Another report described adenomatous and carcinomatous changes in polyps of the small intestine (26).

Juvenile polyp of the stomach usually occurs in hereditary diffuse juvenile polyposis involving the entire digestive tract (27). The polyps are hamartomatous with a prominent stromal component, as distinct from the Peutz-Jeghers polyp, which is dominated by the glandular tissue. Although juvenile polyps are usually not related to carcinoma, there are reports describing adenomatous, dysplastic, and carcinomatous changes in polyps of both stomach and colon (28–30). Similar changes have been observed by the author in a gastric polyp of a patient who had numerous polyps in the stomach and colon.

The fundic gland polyp is composed of a large number of fundic glands covered by normal-appearing superficial mucosa. Fundic gland polyposis apparently occurs mainly in patients with familial polyposis coli (31), but may also occur in patients without the familial syndrome (32). These polyps are not precancerous, but the stomach in the familial cases may contain adenoma, carcinoma, or carcinoid.

RETENTION POLYP

Retention polyps contain dilated glands and abundant stroma that is often chronically inflamed. The glands are hyperplastic to a varying degree. This type of polyp is seen sporadically and in the Cronkhite-Canada syndrome. Sometimes the polyp is made of many dilated glands without inflammation or other reaction (6, 14). These polyps have no known malignant potential.

DISCUSSION

Adenomas, being composed of dysplastic neoplastic cells, are clearly precancerous. Carcinoma develops in any part of the polyp. Treatment must be aimed at total removal of the tissue, surgically if necessary. Smaller polyps may be successfully treated by endoscopic polypectomy (14). Adenomas may change size and new adenomas may form, but they do not disappear (14, 22).

Hyperplastic polyp may become cancerous in a minority of cases (around 0.4 percent). Dysplastic or adenomatous change appears to be the intermediate stage, which occurs in about 5 percent of cases. Without such changes the polyp remains benign. Follow-up endoscopic examinations have shown that most of these polyps remain stationary, although some may disappear and new ones may form (14, 18). After polypectomy they may recur (33), so that regular follow-up is advised (14).

Independent carcinoma may be present in the polyp-bearing stomach, whatever the nature of the polyp. The incidence is lower than in earlier reports—only 3.4 percent of adenoma cases and 4.5 percent of hyperplastic polyp cases in the series reported by Luxén et al. (13).

Malignant change in the polyp has been confirmed for hyperplastic, Peutz-Jeghers, and possibly juvenile polyps. Cancer forms when the polyp develops foci of dysplastic or adenomatous lesions, further indicating the precancerous nature of dysplasia.

The differential diagnosis among the polyps is usually not a problem. There are, however, resemblances among hyperplastic, juvenile, retention, and inflammatory polyps. They are differentiated mainly by the relative amount of glandular and stromal tissue. The degree of hyperplasia of glandular elements decreases in the order above, with no hyperplasia in the inflammatory polyp. In the retention polyp the glands are much dilated and hyperplasia is limited. The terms "retention polyp" and "juvenile polyp" have been used interchangeably for the colon. This is true for isolated colonic polyps. In juvenile polyposis the gastric polyps may have rather prominent hyperplasia of foveolae similar to that in the hyperplastic polyp. There are, however, no aggregates of pyloric glands or prominent muscle bundles. The connective tissue may appear immature even in the absence of inflammatory cells.

Lastly, endoscopic biopsy may not give the correct diagnosis as shown by Seifert and Elster (34). They found a discrepancy in the diagnosis of 53 of 75 polyps. Therefore, total excision of the polyp either endoscopically or surgically is the best way to ascertain the diagnosis as well as to treat the patient.

REFERENCES

1. Rieniets, J. H., and Broders, A. C. Gastric adenomas: A pathological study. *West. J. Surg. Obstet. Gynecol.* 53 (1945):163–170; 54 (1946):21–39.

2. Morson, B. C. Gastric polyps composed of intestinal epithelium. *Br. J. Cancer* 9 (1955):550–557.
3. Ming, S.-C., and Goldman, H. Gastric polyps: A histogenetic classification and its relation to carcinoma. *Cancer* 18 (1965):721–726.
4. Tomasulo, J. Gastric polyps; histologic types and their relationship to gastric carcinoma. *Cancer* 27 (1971):1346–1355.
5. Nakamura, T. Histopathological classification of gastric polyp and its malignant change. *Recent Adv. Gastroenterol.* 1 (1967):477–480.
6. Elster, K. Histologic classification of gastric polyps. *Curr. Top. Pathol.* 65 (1976):77–93.
7. Koch, H. K., Lesch, R., Cremer, M., and Oehlert, W. Polyp and polypoid foveolar hyperplasia in gastric biopsy specimens and the precancerous prevalence. *Front. Gastrointest. Res.* 4 (1979):183–191.
8. Ming, S.-C. The classification and significance of gastric polyps. In *The Gastrointestinal Tract*, edited by Yardley, J. H., and Morson, B. C., pp. 149–175. Baltimore: Williams and Wilkins, 1977.
9. Oota, K., and Sobin, L. H. Histological typing of gastric and oesophageal tumours. International histological classification of tumours. No. 18, p. 37. Geneva: WHO, 1977.
10. Sugano, H., Nakamura, K., and Takagi, K. An atypical epithelium of the stomach. A clinicopathological entity. *Gann Monogr. Cancer Res.* 11 (1971):257–269.
11. Nagayo, T. Histological diagnosis of biopsied gastric mucosa with special reference to that of borderline lesions. *Gann Monogr. Cancer Res.* 11 (1971): 245–256.
12. Fukuchi, S., Hiyama, M., and Mochizucki, T. Endoscopic diagnosis of IIa-subtype of polypoid lesions which belong to borderline lesions between benignancy and malignancy. *Stomach Intest.* 10 (1975):1487–1493.
13. Laxén, F., Sipponen, P., Ihämaki, T., Hakkiluoto, A., and Dortscheva, Z. Gastric polyps; their morphological and endoscopical characteristics and relation to gastric carcinoma. *Acta Pathol. Microbiol. Scand. (A)* 90 (1982):221–228.
14. Rösch, W. Epidemiology, pathogenesis, diagnosis, treatment of benign gastric tumours. *Front. Gastrointest. Res.* 6 (1980):167–184.
15. Nagayo, T. Precursors of human gastric cancer: Their frequencies and histological characteristics. In *Pathophysiology of Carcinogenesis in Digestive Organs*, edited by Farber, E., pp. 151–161. Tokyo: University of Tokyo Press, 1977.
16. Yamagata, S., and Hisamichi, S. Precancerous lesions of the stomach. *World J. Surg.* 3 (1979):671–673.
17. Kozuka, S., Masamoto, K., Suzuki, S., Kubota, K., and Yokoyama, Y. Histogenetic types and size of polypoid lesions in the stomach, with special reference to cancerous change. *Gann* 68 (1977):267–274.
18. Mizuno, H., Kobayashi, S., and Kasugai, T. Endoscopic follow-up of gastric polyps. *Gastrointest. Endosc.* 21 (1975):112–115.
19. Kawai, K., Kizu, M., and Miyaoka, T. Epidemiology and pathogenesis of gastric cancer. *Front. Gastrointest. Res.* 6 (1980):71–86.
20. Remmele, W., and Kolb, E. F. Malignant transformation of hyperplasiogenic polyps of the stomach. Case report. *Endoscopy* 10 (1978):63–65.
21. Ostentag, H., and Georgii, A. Early gastric cancer: A morphologic study of 144 cases. *Pathol. Res. Pract.* 164 (1979):294–315.

22. Kamiya, T., Morishita, T., Asakura, H., Miura, S., Munakata, Y., and Tsuchiya, M. Long term follow-up on gastric adenoma and its relation to gastric protruded carcinoma. *Cancer* 50 (1982):2493–2503.
23. Oehlert, W., Keller, P., Henke, M., and Strauch, M. Gastric mucosal dysplasia: What is its clinical significance? *Front. Gastrointest. Res.* 4 (1979):173–182.
24. Riemann, J. F., Schmidt, H., and Hermanek, P. On the ultrastructure of the gastric "borderline lesion." *J. Cancer Res. Clin. Oncol.* 105 (1983):285–291.
25. Cochet, B., Carrol, J., Desbeillets, L., and Widgren, S. Peutz-Jeghers syndrome associated with gastrointestinal carcinoma. *Gut* 20 (1979):169–175.
26. Perzin, K. H., and Bridge, M. F. Adenomatous and carcinomatous changes in hamartomatous polyps of the small intestine (Peutz-Jeghers syndrome): Report of a case and review of the literature. *Cancer* 49 (1982):971–983.
27. Sachatello, C. R., and Griffen, W. O., Jr. Hereditary polypoid diseases of the gastrointestinal tract; A working classification. *Am. J. Surg.* 129 (1975):198–203.
28. Beacham, D. H., Shields, H. M., Raffensperger, E. C., and Enterline, H. T. Juvenile and adenomatous gastrointestinal polyposis. *Am. J. Dig. Dis.* 23 (1978): 1137–1143.
29. Grigioni, W. F., Alampi, G., Martinelli, G., and Piccoluga, A. Atypical juvenile polyposis. *Histopathology* 5 (1981):361–376.
30. Mills, S. E., and Fechner, R. E. Unusual adenomatous polyps in juvenile polyposis coli. *Am. J. Surg. Pathol.* 6 (1982):177–183.
31. Watanabe, H., Enjoji, M., Yao, T., and Ohsato, K. Gastric lesions in familial adenomatosis coli. Their incidence and histological analysis. *Hum. Pathol.* 9 (1978):269–283.
32. Tatsuta, M., Okuda, S., Tamura, H., and Taniguschi, H. Gastric hamartomatous polyps in the absence of familial polyposis coli. *Cancer* 45 (1980):818–823.
33. Seifert, E. Late results in polypectomy from esophagus and stomach. In *Operative Endoscopy,* edited by Demling, L., and Koch, H. K., pp. 167–171. Stuttgart: Schattauer, 1979.
34. Seifert, E., and Elster, K. Gastric polypectomy. *Am. J. Gastroenterol.* 63 (1975):451–456.

19 HISTOGENESIS OF HUMAN GASTRIC CANCER—WITH SPECIAL REFERENCE TO THE SIGNIFICANCE OF ADENOMA AS A PRECANCEROUS LESION

T. Hirota, T. Okada, M. Itabashi,
and H. Kitaoka

The outstanding advances in endoscopic and radiographic examinations of the digestive tract have led to the feeling that the present methodology for the diagnosis of gastric lesions has been almost perfected. With the invention and improvement of instruments, a large volume of cases has been detected and studied, and the resultant accumulation of experience has yielded a fairly high degree of accuracy in the qualitative and quantitative diagnosis of lesions from X-ray and endoscopic findings.

Accurate preoperative differentiation between benign and malignant gastric lesions has become increasingly necessary in light of the recent conclusion that the malignant development that was hitherto thought to occur in peptic ulcers, hyperplastic polyps, etc., is, in fact, extremely rare.

The improvement of endoscopic instruments has made biopsy much easier and has led to the present widespread use of endoscopic biopsy. This means of histological diagnosis has become absolutely indispensable for the detection of minute cancers, with the ultimate objective of catching gastric cancer in the earliest stage. Histological diagnosis by biopsy can often be conclusively secured, but indeterminable cases also occur occasionally, because it is not always easy to derive an understanding of the whole of a lesion from a miniscule specimen of tissue taken from one part of it. Even for a pathologist this requires long years of experience accumulated from a large volume of cases, as well as the ability to interpret endoscopic and X-ray findings.

The number of reliable gastrointestinal pathologists has not kept pace with the rapid spread of endoscopic biopsy, and there has been a consequent increase in trouble over histopathological diagnosis (1). Most of this trouble concerns regenerative atypia, adenoma, and carcinomatous atypia, especially adenoma. One particular problem is the "overdiagnosis" of adenoma as carcinoma, or else the underdiagnosis of well-differentiated tubular adenocarcinoma as adenoma. The histological diagnosis of adenoma by biopsy is difficult even for gastrointestinal pathologists, and it is not always categorized in the same way. Indeed, adenoma has been variously called atypical epithelium, IIa subtype, adenoma, and other names in Japan. In addition, with the recent introduction of the concept of dysplasia (2,3), the debate over adenoma now involves regenerative atypia and carcinomatous atypia.

Based on our empirical findings, this chapter deals with the various problems involved with adenoma, including its diagnosis by endoscopy, X-ray, and histological biopsy.

MATERIALS AND METHODS

Over the 19 years since the foundation of the National Cancer Center (from May 1962 to December 1980), 144 lesions in 121 cases have been diagnosed as adenoma from 4,163 resected stomachs. Based on these cases, an investigation was conducted into the clinicopathological characteristics of adenoma, the development of malignancy, etc. Many of the specimens were resected for gastric cancer, and therefore most of the adenomas came in the form of multiple lesions. Adenoma found as one of the multiple lesions cannot be treated from the same histogenetic standpoint as uncombined single lesions. But this problem cannot be resolved under the present system in which a solitary adenoma is endoscopically followed up without surgical resection in most cases, while the adenoma associated with carcinoma is resected along with the cancer.

RESULTS

Age and Sex Distribution

The age range of the 121 cases was 37 to 90 years old, with the peak in the sixth decade (Figure 19-1). The average of 62.6 years is comparable with that for protruded-type early gastric cancer (60.3 years).

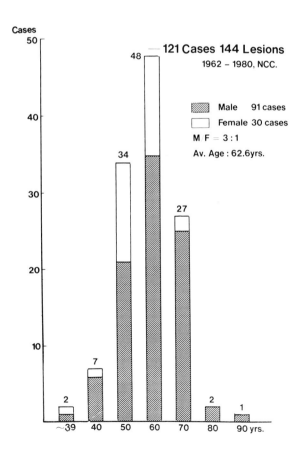

Figure 19-1. Age distribution of the cases of surgically resected stomach with adenoma.

Males outnumbered females by 3:1, a high ratio compared with that for early gastric cancer cases. However, since many of these specimens were resected only because they were combined with gastric cancer, one can hardly say that these figures are purely representative of adenoma. Indeed, if one takes only the 23 uncombined lesions of adenoma, the figures are significantly different, with an average age of 58.3 years and a male-to-female ratio of 13:10.

Combined Lesions

Table 19-1 shows the various types of lesions with which adenoma was combined. Twenty-three cases (25 lesions) were instances of uncombined adenoma. In 13 cases (14 lesions) adenoma was combined with benign lesions, whereas in 55 cases (73 lesions) it was combined with early gastric cancer. Given that the total number of early gastric cancer cases over the same period was 1,072, the proportion of those combined with adenoma is 5.1 percent. There were 29 cases (31 lesions) combined with advanced gastric cancer. One case (one lesion) was combined with leiomyosarcoma. If one makes a division at the year 1972 when endoscopic biopsy became routine, the proportion of cases combined with gastric cancer, especially early cancer, increases significantly. It is possible that there are some differences in clinicopathological characteristics between the combined lesions obtained from surgically resected materials and the uncombined lesions followed up endoscopically without surgical resection. Uncombined cases of adenoma are sometimes resected, but usually only if the lesion exceeds a specified size and histologically shows papillary fea-

Table 19-1. Surgical Materials Containing Adenoma of the Stomach
(121 Cases, 144 Lesions)

Lesions Associated with Adenoma	Total No. of Cases	Total No. of Lesions	Total % of Cases	1962–72		1973–80	
				No. of Cases	No. of Lesions	No. of Cases	No. of Lesions
None	23	25	19.0	14	15	9	10
Early gastric cancer	55	73	45.5	20	27	35	46
Advanced gastric cancer	29	31	24.0	16	17	13	14
Leiomyosarcoma	1	1	0.8			1	1
Benign lesions	13	14	10.7	13	14		
Polyp	3	3					
Gastritis Verrucosa	4	4					
Ulcer	6	6					
Total	121	144	100.0	63	73	58	71

Cases seen at the National Cancer Center, Tokyo, Japan.

tures, since such lesions are difficult to diagnose with any certainty merely by biopsy.

Location of Adenoma

Figure 19-2 shows the frequency of various locations for the 144 lesions following the official Japanese classification (4), dividing the stomach into area C for the upper third, M for the middle third, and A for the lower third. Locations in the M and A areas were very frequent, but extremely rare in the C area. In contrast, when a gastric lesion is detected in association with familial polyposis coli, it often takes the form of a fundic gland polyp and is located in the upper corpus. If one adds to this the fact that intestinal metaplasia tends to develop in the antrum, the interesting location pattern of adenoma may be related to its histogenesis.

Macroscopic Types of Adenoma

Table 19-2 classifies adenoma into macroscopic types corresponding to those of early gastric cancer. For convenience, the type I-like protruded type is divided into the pedunculated type (Ip) and sessile type (Is). As has been pointed out for some time, the most frequent type is

(Text continues on page 241)

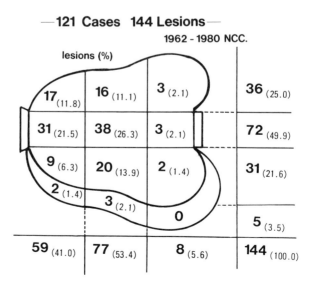

Figure 19-2. Location of the adenoma in surgically resected stomachs.

Table 19-2. Macroscopic Types of Adenoma and Coincidence with
Carcinoma of the Stomach (121 Cases, 144 Lesions)

Macroscopic Types	No. of Lesions (%)	Coincidence with Carcinoma No. of Lesions	%
Is-like ⌒	12 (8.3)	6	50.0
Ip-like ⌒	1 (0.7)	0	0
IIa-like ⌐⌐	99 (68.8)	17	17.2
IIb-like —	18 (12.5)	3	16.7
IIc-like ⌣	8 (5.5)	2	25.0
IIa- + IIc-like ⌣	6 (4.2)	2	33.3
Total	144 (100.0)	30	20.8

Cases seen from 1962 to 1980 at the National Cancer Center, Tokyo, Japan.

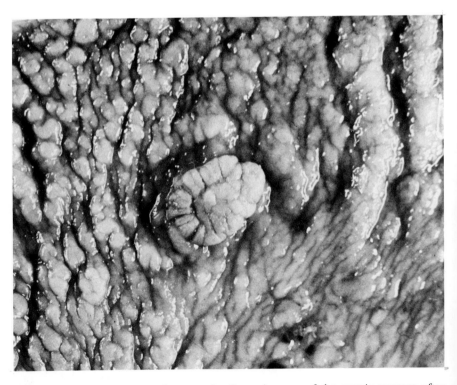

Figure 19-3. Macroscopic photograph of an adenoma of the gastric mucosa after fixation. The flat, elevated, IIa-like lesion is seen in the center of the photograph.

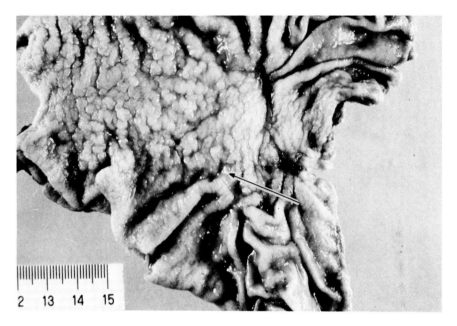

Figure 19-4. Macroscopic photograph of a focus of depressed, IIc-like adenoma (*arrow*) coexisting with multiple ulcers in a surgically resected stomach.

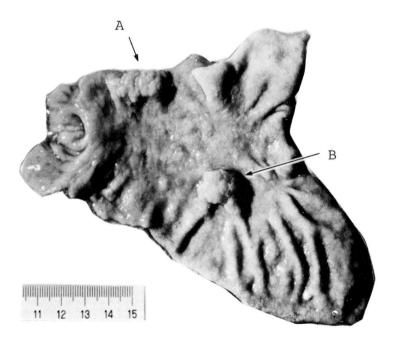

Figure 19-5. Macroscopic photograph of two adenomas (A and B). Lesion B was associated with a microfocus of carcinoma in the same lesion.

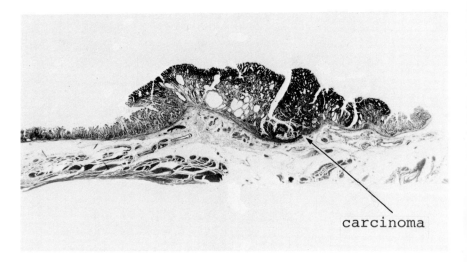

carcinoma

Figure 19-6.   Scanning power view of the section taken from lesion B in Figure 19-5, showing a focus of microcarcinoma (*arrow*) at the center of the adenoma.

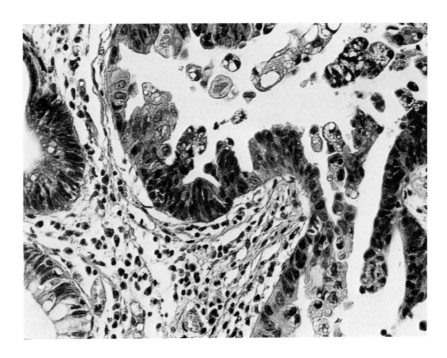

Figure 19-7.   High-power view of the focus of microcarcinoma shown in Figure 19-6. H&E stain. × 320.

the IIa-like flat elevated type, whereas the depressed types are uncommon (Figures 19-3 and 19-4).

The frequency of coincidence with cancer was 20.8 percent (30 lesions). Dividing the macroscopic types, the Is type showed the highest coincidence at 50 percent, whereas the IIa-like lesions had a much lower incidence (Figures 19-5 to 19-7). In five lesions the cancer was located at the center of an adenoma, suggesting a causal relationship between the two. In other lesions the adenomatous component was either adjacent to or inside a carcinoma.

Sizes of Lesions

Figure 19-8 tabulates the lesions by their greatest diameters and gives the corresponding coincidence with cancer. The greater part of the total (80.6 percent, 116 lesions) was taken up by lesions of less than 2 centimeters.

As for the coincidence of cancer within the lesion (Figures 19-9 and 19-10), those larger than 2 centimeters showed a high rate (67.9 percent, 19 of 28) in comparison with those under 2 centimeters (9.5 percent, 11 of 116). This result backs up the current supposition that if a lesion is larger than 2 centimeters, then there is a high probability of cancer within the lesion, even if it has been diagnosed as adenoma.

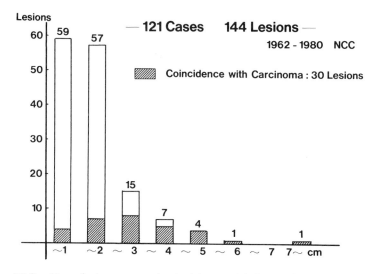

Figure 19-8.   Size of adenomas and coincidence with focus of carcinoma in the same lesions.

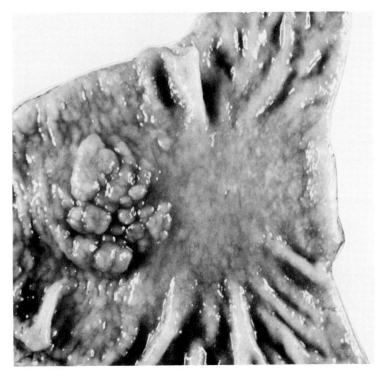

Figure 19-9.   Macroscopic photograph of a clustered type of adenoma with a focus of microcarcinoma in the same lesion. The lesion is 4.8 centimeters in the maximum diameter.

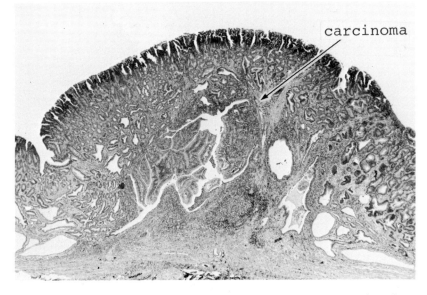

Figure 19-10.   Low-power view of a focus of carcinoma (*arrow*) in the adenoma shown in Figure 19-9. H&E stain. × 40.

Histological Types

In the World Health Organization (WHO) classification (5), adenoma is divided into three subtypes—tubular, papillary, and papillotubular. Most of the 144 lesions were tubular adenomas (as many as 107 lesions, 74.3 percent), followed by papillotubular adenoma (33 lesions, 22.9 percent); papillary adenoma was very rare (4 instances, 2.8 percent) (Table 19-3).

Of 107 lesions of tubular adenoma only 15 (14 percent) were coincident with cancer within the same lesion, whereas by contrast the coincidence rates for the papillotubular and papillary forms were 36.4 (12 of 33) and 75 (3 of 4) percent, respectively. Thus, lesions showing papillary features tend to have a high coincidence with cancer in the same lesion.

Histological Atypia

By the criteria shown in Table 19-4, we have divided histological atypia into grades I, II, and III. As shown in Table 19-5, 44 lesions (30.6 percent) were of grade I, 79 (54.8 percent) of grade II, and 21 (14.6 percent) of grade III (Figures 19-11 to 19-13).

Grades I and II showed roughly the same cancer coincidence rate (15.9 and 16.5 percent, respectively), but the rate for grade III was comparatively high at 47.6 percent (10 of 21).

Table 19-3. Histological Classification of Adenoma and Coincidence with Carcinoma of the Stomach (121 Cases, 144 Lesions)

Histological Types	No. of Lesions (%)	Coincidence with Carcinoma	
		No. of Lesions	%
Tubular	107 (74.3)	15	14.0
Papillotubular	33 (22.9)	12	36.4
Papillary	4 (2.8)	3	75.0
Total	144 (100.0)	30	20.8

Cases seen from 1962 to 1980 at the National Cancer Center, Tokyo, Japan.

Table 19-4. Histological Features of Regenerative Atypia, Adenoma, and Well-Differentiated Adenocarcinoma

	Regenerative Atypia (Benign)	Adenoma			Adenocarcinoma (Well-Differentiated)
		Grade I	Grade II	Grade III	
Nucleus	Large, round	Spindle	Spindle	Spindle, ovoid	Spindle, ovoid
Nuclear/cyto-plasmic ratio	Normal	Almost normal	Increased slightly	Increased moderately	Increased markedly
Nuclear stratification	–	Only in gland base	Slightly from surface to base	Moderately from surface to base	Prominent
Nuclear polarity	Lost, sometimes	Preserved	Preserved	Preserved	Preserved
Intestinal cells					
Goblet cells	+[a]	+	Few/–	–/Rare	–/Rare
Paneth cells	+[a]	+	Few/–	–/Rare	–/Rare
Glandular differentiation	+	+	–	–	–
Structural abnormality	–	–	±	+	+
Transition to adjacent normal mucosa	+	–	–	–	–
Biopsy diagnosis	Group II		Group III	Borderline lesion	Group V

–, Absent; +, present.
[a]Applies only to metaplastic mucosa.

Table 19-5. Histological Atypia of Adenoma and Coincidence with
Carcinoma of the Stomach (121 Cases, 144 Lesions)

Histological Atypia	No. of Lesions (%)	Coincidence with Carcinoma	
		No. of Lesions	%
Grade I	44 (30.6)	7	15.9
Grade II	79 (54.8)	13	16.5
Grade III	21 (14.6)	10	47.6
Total	144 (100.0)	30	20.8

Cases seen from 1962 to 1980 at the National Cancer Center, Tokyo, Japan.

Incidence of "Gastric-Type" Adenoma

Recently, Kato et al. (6) have proposed the term "gastric-type adenoma" for lesions that show villous features consisting of cells similar to the normal foveolar epithelia (Figure 19-14) and that show

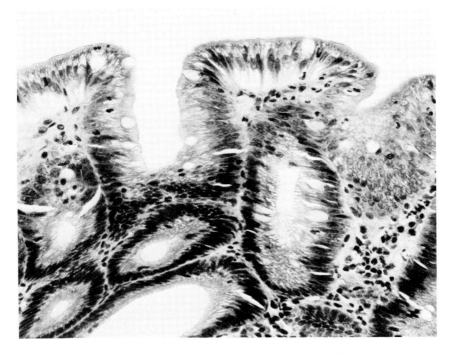

Figure 19-11.   Photomicrograph of a tubular adenoma with slight atypia (grade I). H&E stain. × 200.

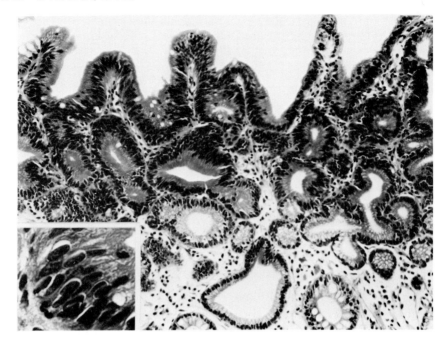

Figure 19-12.   Photomicrograph of a tubular adenoma with moderate atypia (grade II). H&E stain. × 100; × 1,400 (inset).

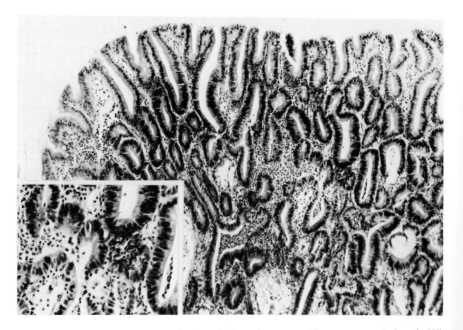

Figure 19-13.   Photomicrograph of a tubular adenoma with severe atypia (grade III). H&E stain. × 100; × 2,400 (inset).

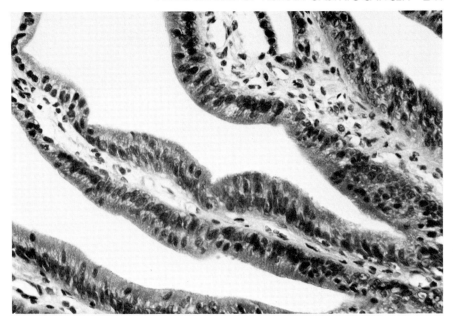

Figure 19-14. Photomicrograph of a gastric-type villous adenoma with moderate atypia (grade II). H&E stain. × 200.

pale abundant cytoplasm without goblet or Paneth cells. A lesion with these special features has a character similar to gastric epithelium, not only in the surface pattern of mucosubstances, but also in that periodic acid-Schiff staining is positive and alcian blue staining negative. Kato et al. (6) report that gastric-type atypical epithelium (adenoma) is extremely rare and that over 90 percent of atypical epithelium (adenoma) is of the intestinal type. Of the 144 lesions under review, no more than six (4.2 percent) were thought to be of Kato et al.'s gastric type (6). Again, only three lesions (2.1 percent) were thought to be of a mixed gastric/intestinal type. Most (93.7 percent) of the lesions were of the so-called intestinal-type atypical epithelium (adenoma), which has the characteristics of intestinal epithelium.

Of the 135 intestinal-type lesions, a surprisingly small number (26 lesions, 19.3 percent) were coincident with cancer when compared with the gastric type (4 of 6 lesions, 66.7 percent) (Table 19-6).

It is suggested by some that the gastric type of adenoma is an extremely well-differentiated carcinoma, but much more research on this is thought to be necessary. For the present, however, what can be said is that the gastric type has a high cancer coincidence rate, whereas the common intestinal type of adenoma has an extremely low rate. From the point of view of gastric cancer in general, the role of gastric-type adenoma as a precancerous lesion is small.

Table 19-6. Histological Subclassification of Adenoma of the Stomach
(121 Cases, 144 Lesions)

| Type of Adenoma | No. of Lesions | % | Coincidence with Carcinoma | |
			No. of Lesions	%
Gastric type	6	4.2	4	66.7
Mixed type	3	2.1	0	0
Intestinal type	135	93.7	26	19.3
Total	144	100.0	30	20.8

Cases seen from 1962 to 1980 at the National Cancer Center, Tokyo, Japan.

DISCUSSION

In Japan the term "atypical epithelium" is widely used, but it is hard to define accurately. Indeed, there is no settled view among pathologists as to its true identity or its etiology. Generally speaking, atypical epithelium has a group of atypical glands that occupy a specific area and that differ from clear regenerative atypia and carcinomatous atypia. For some time it has been referred to as atypical epithelium, IIa subtype, Nakamura type III polyp, adenoma, etc., but the basic point is that it is a type of lesion hard to distinguish from well-differentiated tubular adenocarcinoma.

Since adenoma usually takes the macroscopic form of a small protrusion, it has been treated as having the quality of a polyp. For instance, in 1962 Nakamura et al. (7) classified it as a type III polyp on the grounds of its histological characteristics. In 1965 it was classified by Ming (8) as an adenomatous polyp, and thus began to attract attention as a discrete type of stomach polyp. In Japan adenoma is distinguished from a polyp on the ground that polyps are benign inflammatory lesions, whereas we tend to treat adenoma as a benign/malignant borderline lesion. Strictly speaking, however, a true borderline lesion is one that cannot be histologically judged benign or malignant at all, whereas adenoma is mostly benign in nature. The term "benign/malignant borderline lesion" must therefore be used in a broader sense when applied to the adenoma.

As has been known for some time, the most common age group for the development of adenoma is the same as that for gastric cancer, and its favored locations are the middle and lower third regions of the stomach. As suggested by its alternative name, IIa subtype (9), the macroscopic form is seen as a IIa-like protrusion in nearly 70 percent of cases. Since protruded lesions in general amounted to 77.8 percent of all lesions reported, we are not surprised to find that adenoma frequently appears in a protruded form.

With regard to macroscopic form, the flat IIb-like and the depressed IIc-like forms are of interest: The IIb-like form is very rarely diagnosed preoperatively, but is usually a minute lesion discovered by chance in the course of postoperative histopathological examination. Since IIb-like lesions are so very small and have a low rate of coincidence with cancer within the lesion, it is thought that this might possibly be an early form of atypical epithelium. On the other hand, the IIc- and IIa + IIc-like forms made up 9.6 percent of the total, and the cancer coincidence rate was second only to the Is form.

Considering the high rate of coincidence with cancer of lesions of over 2 centimeters, sessile type I-like lesions, and depressed lesions, it is clearly necessary to conduct further detailed examination of these lesions even after the material collected by endoscopic biopsy has been diagnosed as adenoma. Further, in cases with lesions showing a papillary feature, grade III atypia, or Kato et al.'s gastric-type adenoma (6), we consider strongly the possibility of coincident cancer.

There is still no conclusion as to the question of whether adenoma is a neoplastic or nonneoplastic lesion. Ming (8) classed adenomatous polyps as neoplastic. When Nakamura and Nakano (10) introduced the term "type III polyp," they held it to be neoplastic with a high potential for becoming malignant; but in light of detailed examination of its two-layered structure, they now disfavor this view. On examining the histogenesis of minute adenoma, Nakamura et al. (11) reported that it may be either a neoplasm or an incipient type of intestinal metaplasia of the gastric mucosa.

The WHO treats what we often call atypical epithelium as neoplastic, classifying it as adenoma. We hold the same view, since the tubular glands show an atypia that can hardly be considered malignant and occupy a specific localized area that has a clear frontier with the normal tissue. We also follow the WHO histological classification into the three types—tubular, papillary, and papillotubular adenoma.

In the large intestine, the process of changing from adenoma to carcinoma is already established as the adenoma-carcinoma sequence, but in the stomach only 5 of 1,000 early gastric cancer cases treated at the National Cancer Center could be said to have focal cancer in adenoma, i.e., a clearly malignant development in the adenoma. An extended follow-up study of adenoma for up to 5 years with X-ray and endoscopy revealed no significant growth or malignant development (9, 12, 13). However, in light of the results of our present survey that 20.8 percent of the adenomas were accompanied by cancer, some connection with cancer must be considered. There are two possible explanations for the coexistence of adenoma and carcinoma within the same lesion: either the two components originally developed separately, but then merged together as the lesions grew; or part of the adenoma became malignant. When the latter is the case, the lesion can be caught in an early form as focal cancer in adenoma.

The fact that adenoma shows a preference for the same location as differentiated adenocarcinoma suggests that even when the two coexist in the same lesion, there is still the possibility that they originally developed separately. The survey of Kato et al. (6) reveals that of 34 stomachs resected for atypical epithelium (adenoma), only 5 cases (14.7 percent) showed amalgamation with a minute carcinoma smaller than 5 millimeters. In the present survey the frequency of malignant development in adenoma lay between 20.8 percent (30 lesions with coexisting cancer) and 3.5 percent (5 lesions with cancer in the center of an adenoma).

From examination of the background mucosa of minute lesions, we have found that adenoma and differentiated adenocarcinoma are often accompanied by incomplete intestinal metaplasia in the background mucosa (14–16). In contrast, in the case of hyperplastic polyp, which very rarely becomes malignant and is thought to be due to regenerative changes, incomplete intestinal metaplasia was hardly ever found in its background (17).

SUMMARY

The clinicopathological aspects of 144 gastric adenomas and their significance as precancerous lesions were studied. The results and our conclusions are summarized below.

Cases were concentrated in the older age groups, peaking in the sixth decade. The overall male-to-female ratio was 3:1, but among cases of pure and simple adenoma, it was nearly equal at 1.3:1.

Most lesions were located in the M and A regions, whereas those in the C region were rare.

Lesions were of an elevated type in 77.8 percent, and IIa-like elevations were especially frequent.

Most (80.6 percent) of the lesions were less than 2 centimeters in diameter, with 41 percent smaller than 1 centimeter and 39.6 percent between 1 and 2 centimeters.

Focal cancer in adenoma, or what is held to be malignant development of adenoma, was found in at least 5 lesions (3.5 percent); however, there were 30 lesions that combined the two elements of adenoma and carcinoma within the same lesion (i.e., the cancer coincidence rate was 20.8 percent). It is therefore concluded that the real frequency of malignant development of adenoma lies between 3.5 and 20.8 percent.

From the macroscopic point of view, the main factors associated with high cancer coincidence are: a size larger than 2 centimeters; and a lesion of the Is form or of a depressed type. From the histological point of view, associated factors are: papillary features; grade III atypia; and the so-called "gastric-type" adenoma.

ACKNOWLEDGMENTS

The authors are greatly indebted to Dr. Y. Shimosato, Chief of the Pathology Division of the National Cancer Center Research Institute, Tokyo, and Mr. Alexander Scott for their helpful suggestions and reading of the manuscript. We thank Mrs. S. Matsuoka and Miss Y. Yamauchi for their skillful technical assistance. We are also obliged to the members of the gastrointestinal tract-study group of the National Cancer Center Hospital.

This work was supported in part by Grants-in-Aid for Cancer Research from the Ministry of Education (grant no. 7010067).

REFERENCES

1. Hirota, T., Itabashi, M., Unagami, M., and Oguro, Y. Accuracy of histopathological diagnosis by endoscopical biopsy specimens of the stomach [Japanese]. *J. Therapy* 64 (1982):317–327.
2. Morson, B. C., Sobin, L. H., Grundmann, E., Johansen, A., Nagayo, T., and Serck-Hanssen, A. Precancerous condition and epithelial dysplasia in the stomach. *J. Clin. Pathol.* 33 (1980):711–721.
3. Cuello, C., Correa, P., Zarama, G., Lopez, J., Murray, J., and Gordillo, G. Histopathology of gastric dysplasia; correlations with gastric juice chemistry. *Am. J. Surg. Pathol.* 3 (1979):491–500.
4. Japanese Research Society for Gastric Cancer. *The General Rules for the Gastric Cancer Study in Surgery and Pathology.* Tokyo: Kanehara Publishing Co., Inc., 1979.

5. Oota, K. Histological typing of gastric and esophageal tumours. International Histological Classification of Tumours, No. 18, p. 19. Geneva: World Health Organization, 1977.

6. Kato, H., Yanagisawa, A., and Sugano, H. Borderline lesion of the stomach [Japanese]. *Saishin-Igaku* 36 (1981):21–30.

7. Nakamura, T., Iwamaru, M., and Takekawa, K. Pathology of gastric polyp [Japanese]. *J. Jpn. Surg. Soc.* 63 (1962):949–951.

8. Ming, S.-C. Gastric polyps; a histogenetic classification and its relation to cancer *Cancer* 18 (1965):721–726.

9. Fukuchi, S., and Mochizuki, T. Significance of endoscopical biopsy for the diagnosis of protruded lesions of the stomach [Japanese]. *Gastroenterol. Endosc.* 9 (1967):105–107.

10. Nakamura, T., and Nakano, G. Problem of gastric adenoma [Japanese]. *Jpn. J. Clin. Med.* 34 (1976):1368–1377.

11. Nakamura, K., Sugano, H., Takagi, K., and Kumakura, K. Histogenesis of atypical epithelial lesions of the stomach—Light and electron-microscopic study with special reference to micro-focus of atypical epithelium [Japanese]. *Jpn. J. Cancer Clin.* 15 (1969):955–969.

12. Takezawa, H. Studies on the gastric atypical epithelium: Comparison of it with early gastric cancer type IIa [English summary]. *Gastroenterol. Endosc.* 15 (1973):375–388.

13. Sakamoto, K. A long-term follow-up study of gastric polyps [English summary]. *Fukuoka Acta Med.* 71 (1980):558–573.

14. Matsukura, N., Suzuki, K., Kawachi, T., Aoyagi, M., Sugimura, T., Kitaoka, H., Numajiri, H., Shirota, A., Itabashi, M., and Hirota, T. Distribution of marker enzymes and mucin in intestinal metaplasia in human stomach and relation of complete and incomplete type of intestinal metaplasia to minute gastric carcinomas. *J. Natl. Cancer Inst.* 65 (1980):231–240.

15. Yoshida, H., Hirota, T., Itabashi, M., Misaka, R., Onuma, C., Unagami, M., Oguro, Y., Yoshimori, M., Kitaoka, H., Hirata, K., Kawachi, T., and Matsukura, N. Spatial relation between gastric carcinoma and subtype of intestinal metaplasia [English summary]. *Prog. Dig. Endosc.* 17 (1980):120–124.

16. Onuma, C., Hirota, T., Itabashi, M., Misaka, R., Yoshida, H., Unagami, M., Oguro, Y., Yoshimori, M., Kitaoka, H., Kawachi, T., and Matsukura, N. Spatial relation between gastric atypical epithelium and subtype of intestinal metaplasia [English summary]. *Prog. Dig. Endosc.* 17 (1980):115–119.

17. Okada, T., Hirota, T., Unagami, M., Itabashi, M., Oonishi, T., Higo, M., Oguro, Y., Kitaoka, H., Hirata, K., Kawachi, T., and Matsukura, N. Spatial relation between hyperplastic polyp and subtypes of intestinal metaplasia [English summary]. *Prog. Dig. Endosc.* 18 (1981):108–111.

20 GASTRIC POLYPOID LESIONS AND THEIR SIGNIFICANCE AS CANCER PRECURSORS

G. Zampi and M. L. Carcangiu

Although there is general agreement concerning the histogenesis and nomenclature of intestinal polyps and their relation to cancer, there is still controversy regarding these problems with respect to gastric polyps.

TYPES OF GASTRIC POLYPS

Although some authors (1–11) have put forward some interesting alternative suggestions, the textbooks on pathology, the treatises on tumors, and the monographs on gastrointestinal pathology favor, with slight differences of a semantic nature, the traditional classification of gastric polyps (2, 3, 5–7, 12–15).

Since to distinguish on a histological basis between hamartomatous and regenerative polyps is not always easy and is of little practical interest, as is also the identification of a specific category of inflammatory polyps, it is usual to subdivide gastric polyps into two classes: regenerative (hyperplastic) and adenomatous. The former are supposed to be of inflammatory or regenerative origin, and the latter true neoplasms, some of which could contain carcinomatous areas.

The incidence of various types of gastric polyps is not always easy to assess, partly because the data are taken from statistics composed of a limited number of cases, often not entirely reliable because not homogeneous. There is, however, a general agreement that regenerative polyps are much more frequent than those of neoplastic nature.

MALIGNANT POTENTIAL OF GASTRIC POLYPS

As regards the relationship to gastric cancer, it is accepted (1–7, 16) that most common polyps, that is, the regenerative (hyperplastic) ones, have a very low malignant potential and that the adenomatous polyps, on the other hand, have a significant tendency to become malignant.

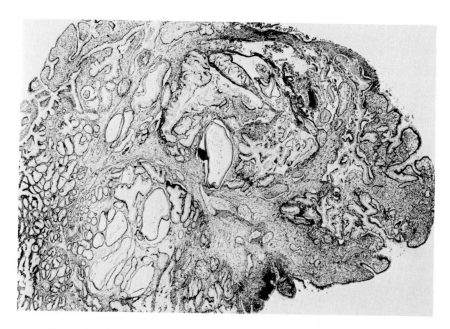

Figure 20-1.   Classic regenerative (hyperplastic) polypoid lesion showing typical foveolar epithelium, edematous stroma, cysts, and interdigitation of smooth muscle with glands. H&E stain. × 14.

Although only adenomatous polyps are usually considered precursors of gastric carcinoma, there is also evidence of the frequent association of cancer with gastric regenerative polyps. Despite this, little importance has been given to polyps as morphological precursors of gastric cancer because all polypoid lesions, and specifically neoplastic polyps, were considered rare. This was held to be so up until a few years ago, because gastric polyps were encountered only through surgery or autopsy. Nowadays, however, owing to the more frequent use of endoscopic polypectomy, they are seen much more frequently.

Therefore, the problem of gastric polyps and their relation to gastric cancer can be studied within a wider context, taking advantage also of the availability of symptomless lesions and tumors in the early stages of their development.

Moreover, in recent years there has been a dramatic improvement in the understanding of hyperplastic-metaplastic lesions of gastric mucosa and particularly of gastric dysplasia as a morphological marker of transition from a simple precancerous condition to an actual precancerous lesion (4, 8, 9, 11, 17).

OUR EXPERIENCE

Looking at the problem from this new perspective, so different from the traditional one, we have tried to evaluate a considerable number of gastric polypoid lesions on file in the Institute of Pathology of the University of Florence, Florence, Italy. We have reviewed only the epithelial polyps and, among them, some with limited carcinomatous areas. We have excluded cancers of mere polypoid appearance.

Two hundred sixty-eight polypoid lesions obtained mainly by endoscopy were the object of our observations.

Assigning the cases to the various subgroups according to the traditional classification, it was found that most (72.7 percent) were of the regenerative type (Figure 20-1), including the seldom-seen forms of fibroinflammatory and hamartomatous polyps (Figure 20-2), and that the "neoplastic" type (Figures 20-3 and 20-4) was considerably rarer (18.2 percent). In addition, it is particularly interesting to observe that in a significant number of cases (9.1 percent), regenerative aspects were present simultaneously with adenomatous changes in the same polypoid lesion (Figure 20-5).

We seldom observed severe atypia in epithelium with the characteristics of superficial (foveolar) epithelium, the dysplastic changes

(Text continues on page 258)

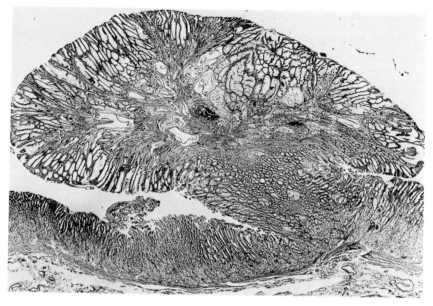

Figure 20-2.   Pedunculated "nonneoplastic" polyp with a mixed pattern, regenerative on the right and hamartomatous on the left. H&E stain. × 8.

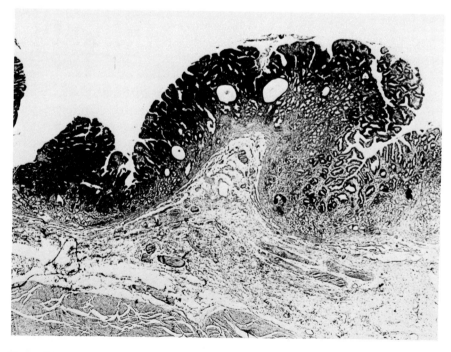

Figure 20-3.   An "adenomatous" gastric lesion with a slightly raised growth pattern. H&E stain. × 16.

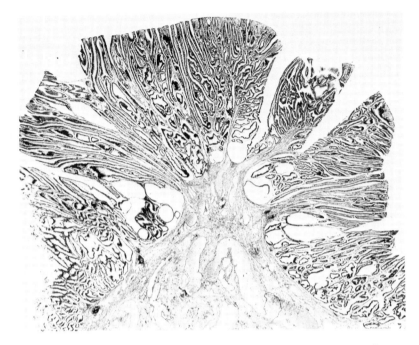

Figure 20-4. Tubulovillous gastric "adenoma." H&E stain. ×9.

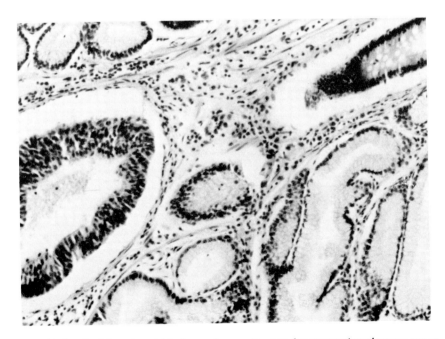

Figure 20-5. In this polypoid lesion, adenomatous and regenerative changes are associated. H&E stain. ×148.

usually being correlated to intestinal metaplasia (Figure 20-6) through the changes of "adenomatous dysplasia" described by Cuello et al. (18). Clear evidence of dysplastic alterations suggestive of potential malignancy were observed in 27 polypoid lesions of the adenomatous type (55.1 percent) and in 11 polyps with simultaneous regenerative and adenomatous features (45.8 percent) (Figure 20-7).

Independent of the type of polyp, the appearance of clearly carcinomatous areas (Figure 20-8) was generally preceded by changes in the gastric epithelium, which assumed an intestinal aspect, possibly but not necessarily showing a polypoid appearance with a tubular, villous, or tubulovillous arrangement.

DISCUSSION

Our present experience indicates that in the majority of cases of so-called gastric polyps, it is inflammation that stimulates the development of protruding lesions. These usually take the classic form of hyperplastic-regenerative "polyps" with typical foveolar epithelium,

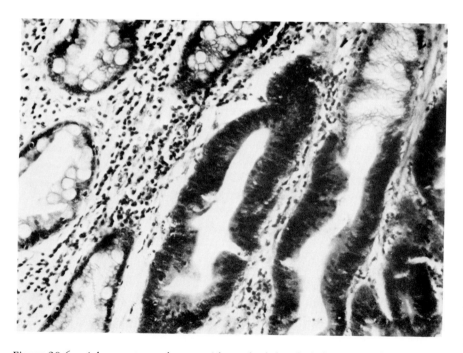

Figure 20-6.   Adenomatous change with marked dysplasia in intestinal metaplasia. H&E stain. × 185.

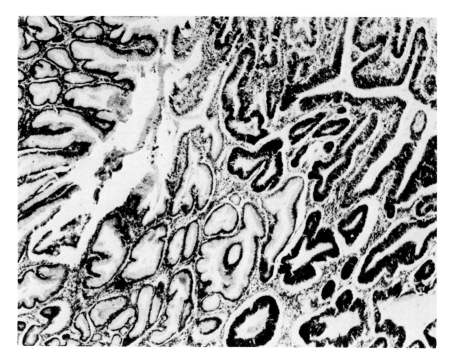

Figure 20-7.   Regenerative change, intestinal metaplasia, and severe adenomatous dysplasia coexist in a gastric polypoid lesion. H&E stain. × 50.

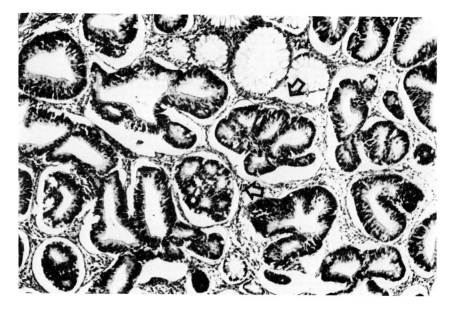

Figure 20-8.   Cancerous change (*arrows*) is seen at the center of a gastric adenomatous polyp. H&E stain. × 50.

dilated glands, edematous stroma, and interdigitation of smooth muscle with glands.

Sometimes, on this inflammatory-regenerative basis, changes of intestinal metaplasia are seen. Later, these progressively tend to increase, so that occasionally the regenerative lesions assume the appearance of a tubular or villous intestinal polyp.

Looking at the origin of the "neoplastic polyps," we see the same process: It is still intestinal metaplasia that gives rise to the "adenomatous" lesion and through pseudostratification and dysplasia to carcinomatous change.

In our opinion there is no such thing as a true benign tumor that transforms itself into a cancer, but rather there are hyperplastic-metaplastic lesions that through dysplasia may become malignant.

The term "polyp" is a conventional one and covers a wide range of lesions that exemplify the many ways in which gastric mucosa reacts to various stimuli. Obviously, the classification of polyps in the traditional subgroups is itself artificial, as is seen from the difficulties found in categorizing some of the cases.

Except for the doubts expressed above concerning the suitability of the term "polyp," our observations agree with the classification of gastric polyps proposed by Nakamura (10) and fully confirm the subdivision proposed by Kozuka et al. (1). The subdivision of the gastric type of polyps into two forms, pure gastric and gastric with metaplasia, is of particular importance, because it links the gastric type (hyperplastic-regenerative) to the metaplastic type and suggests a connection with cancer that falls between the lowest incidence (i.e., that of the gastric type) and the highest (i.e., that of the metaplastic type).

Seen from this perspective, it is not surprising that cancer coexists with hyperplastic (regenerative) polyps, these being a context within which metaplastic-dysplastic changes can occur and give rise to cancer.

We can therefore conclude that the development of "adenomatous" dysplasia, associated or not with the polypoid appearance, may be a possible source of cancer, at least with respect to some carcinomatous lesions of the stomach.

Consequently, for gastric cancer, as for intestinal cancer, we face the same question: namely, whether it occurs through adenomatous polyps or de novo. If we assume that so-called adenomas are in reality metaplastic epithelia with dysplasia and not true benign neoplasms, then we can conclude that the question deals only with semantics rather than a matter of substance. In other words, gastric carcinomas arise in a metaplastic-dysplastic mucosa that may assume the appearance but not the true nature of an adenoma.

REFERENCES

1. Kozuka, S., Masamoto, K., Suzuki, S., Kubota, K., and Yokoyama, Y. Histogenetic types and size of polypoid lesions in the stomach, with special reference to cancerous change. *Gann* 68 (1977):267–274.
2. Lesbros, F., Labadie, M., Truchot, R., and Berger, F. Les polypes gastriques. Essai de classification anatomo-pathologique portant sur 83 polypes. *Arch. Anat. Cytol. Pathol.* 25 (1977):251–257.
3. Ming, S.-C. *Atlas of Tumor Pathology. Tumors of Esophagus and Stomach.* Washington: Armed Forces Institute of Pathology, 1973.
4. Ming, S.-C. Dyplasia of gastric epithelium. *Front. Gastrointest. Res.* 4 (1979):164–172.
5. Ming, S.-C., and Goldman, H. Gastric polyps. A histogenetic classification and its relation to carcinoma. *Cancer* 18 (1965):721–726.
6. Monaco, A. P., Roth, S. I., Castleman, B., and Welch, C. E. Adenomatous polyps of the stomach. A clinical and pathological study of 152 cases. *Cancer* 15 (1962):456–467.
7. Morson, B. C., and Dawson, I. M. P. *Gastrointestinal Pathology*, 2nd ed., pp. 140–147. Oxford: Blackwell Scientific Publications, 1979.
8. Morson, B. C., Sobin, L. H., Grundmann, E., Johansen, A., Nagayo, T., and Serck-Hanssen, A. Precancerous condition and epithelial dysplasia in the stomach. *J. Clin. Pathol.* 33 (1980):711–721.
9. Nagayo, T. Histological diagnosis of biopsied gastric mucosa with special reference to that of borderline lesions. *Gann Monogr. Cancer Res.* 11 (1971): 245–256.
10. Nakamura, T. Histopathological classification of gastric polyp and its malignant change. *Recent Adv. Gastroenterol.* 1 (1967):477–480.
11. Oehlert, W. Biological significance of dysplasias of the epithelium and of atrophic gastritis. In *Gastric Cancer*, edited by Herfarth, Ch., and Schlag, P., pp. 91–104. Berlin: Springer-Verlag, 1979.
12. Berg, J. W. Histological aspects of the relation between gastric adenomatous polyps and cancers. *Cancer* 11 (1958):1149–1155.
13. Tomasulo, J. Gastric polyps. Histological types and their relationship to gastric carcinoma. *Cancer* 27 (1971):1346–1355.
14. Elster, K. Histologic classification of gastric polyps. *Curr. Top. Pathol.* 63 (1977):77–93.
15. Goldman, D. S., and Appelman, H. D. Gastric mucosal polyps. *Am. J. Clin. Pathol.* 58 (1972):434–444.
16. Hermanek, P. Gastric polyps and gastric cancer. In *Gastric Cancer*, edited by Herfarth, Ch., and Schlag, P., pp. 147–148. Berlin: Springer-Verlag, 1979.
17. Grundmann, E., and Schlake, W. Histology of possible precancerous stages in the stomach. In *Gastric Cancer*, edited by Herfarth, Ch., and Schlag, P., pp. 72–82. Berlin: Springer-Verlag, 1979.
18. Cuello, C., Correa, P., Zarama, G., Lopez, J., Murray, J., and Gordillo, G. Histopathology of gastric dysplasias. Correlations with gastric juice chemistry. *Am. J. Surg. Pathol.* 3 (1979):491–500.

VI CHRONIC GASTRIC ULCER

21 RELATIONSHIP BETWEEN GASTRIC CARCINOMA AND CHRONIC GASTRIC ULCER

S.-C. Ming

The precancerous nature of chronic gastric ulcers has been suggested by many reports. A century has passed since Hauser (1–3) began his pathologic studies on the development of gastric cancer in chronic ulcer. Hauser's criteria of ulcer-cancer (3) are still widely used. The term "ulcer-cancer" is applied to a carcinoma that is thought to have arisen in a chronic gastric ulcer according to the following criteria: The ulcer is chronic as evidenced by dense fibrosis disrupting the muscularis propria together with obliterating endarteritis and fusion of the muscularis mucosa with the muscularis propria at the ulcer border (4); and the carcinomatous tissue is present at the margin but not at the base of the ulcer. The ulcer-cancer is therefore, by definition, most likely an early cancer. However, it may also apply to an advanced cancer as long as the base of the ulcer does not contain tumor. In fact, an example illustrated by Hauser (2) clearly had metastasis in the lymph nodes. Thus, many cases reported in the literature appear to include both early and advanced cancers.

The relationship between chronic gastric ulcer and cancer has been a controversial topic for a long time, mostly on the question of the frequency of incidence. Like other precursors of gastric cancer, several aspects of this relationship can now be considered as more information becomes available. These aspects are reviewed in this chapter.

FREQUENCY OF CARCINOMA IN GASTRIC ULCERS

The reported incidences of carcinoma in gastric ulcers vary greatly. Three separate sources of information should be considered: ulcerated cancers, cancer in resected ulcers, and cancer in medically treated ulcers.

Ulcerated Cancers

Gastric carcinoma is often ulcerated. In our material 25 percent of advanced cancers were ulcerated. In some cases the ulcer base is free of tumor. This is not surprising, since the acid-secreting area of the gastric mucosa is relatively normal in many cancerous stomachs. It is unusual, however, that the ulcer destroys all the cancer tissue at the ulcer base. Conversely, an ulcer may become cancerous; then the cancer overtakes the ulcerative process. Thus, the presence or absence of ulceration in an advanced carcinoma imparts no special meaning. Better insights may be gained by evaluating early gastric carcinomas. An early attempt in this regard was made in 1925 by Dible (5) who found 5 ulcer-cancers among 33 early gastric carcinomas. However, only two of these had a long history of cancer.

With the advance in endoscopic diagnosis, many reports on early gastric cancer have been published in the last 20 years, mostly from Japan. In 1963 Oota (6) reported that 85 percent of cancer cases had preexisting ulcer. The figure in Kuru's series (7) was 38 percent and in Sano's series (8) 70 percent. These very high incidences were due partly to a broad usage of the term "ulcer" in Japan as pointed out by Sano (8). For instance, in Sano's cases (8), the ulcer was deep in 25 percent, moderate in 24 percent, and shallow in 51 percent. Even taking this into account, however, the ulcer incidence in early cancer was very high in these early reports. More recently, the importance of chronic ulcer as a precancerous lesion has been downgraded, and Oota (9) no longer considered it an important cancer cause in 1976. There had apparently been a steady decrease in the incidence of deeply ulcerated (Type III) early gastric cancer in Japan as noted by

Nagayo (10): Type III early cancer decreased from nearly 70 percent in 1953 to about 10 percent in 1974 with a corresponding increase of Type IIc (slightly depressed) cancers. More important, cases fulfilling the criteria of ulcer-cancer have decreased from over 1 percent in 1953 to nearly zero percent since 1969. Nagayo (10) also noted that the number of stomachs resected for ulcer had also declined. These data suggest that with better medical management, gastric ulceration has become less common in both benign and malignant situations. It is therefore reasonable to assume that the ulcer in many early carcinomas is secondary. This view was enhanced by the observation of Sakita et al. (11) that the ulcer in ulcerated early cancers might heal in 18 to 25 percent of cases. The healing of malignant ulcer was also noted by Wenger et al. (12).

Cancer in Resected Ulcers

The incidence of cancer in resected ulcers reported in the literature varied from 1 (13) to 6 (14) percent. More recent reports give similar findings. Yamagata and Hisamichi (15) reported an incidence of 2.26 percent in 1979 and Haukland et al. (16) reported 2.6 percent in 1981. As noted by Majima et al. (13), nearly one-half of ulcer-cancer patients had ulcer symptoms for less than 3 years, suggesting a secondary nature of the ulcer. Hirohata (17) noted a slightly higher incidence of gastric cancer than expected in ulcer patients followed for 8 to 18 years, but the difference was not statistically significant.

Cancer in Medically Treated Ulcers

Larson et al. (18) reported in 1961 the discovery of cancer in 48 of 391 ulcer patients followed for 10 to 19 years. In only 16 of these cases, cancer was found 5 or more years after the diagnosis of ulcer, an incidence of 4 percent. The incidence in biopsied cases reported by Thunold and Wetteland (19) was 1.3 percent. In a report in 1980, Kawai et al. (20) gave incidences of 2.2 and 2.3 percent in patients followed for 9 and 15 years, respectively. It was not clear, however, whether the cancer was actually in the ulcer. When this factor was considered, the incidence of cancer in ulcer was lower. For instance, among ulcer patients studied by Montgomery and Richardson (21), three developed carcinoma in 5 years. In two cases the cancer was not in the ulcer. The incidence of cancer in the ulcer was only 0.6 percent (1 of 160 cases). A similar situation was noted earlier by Swynnerton and Tanner (22) in 1953 and led them to conclude that carcinoma and ulcer were unrelated, but might occur in the same type of "degenerate mucosa." This view coincides with the finding by Stemmermann et al. (23) in 1977 that both gastric ulcer and gastric cancer tend to occur in the area of intestinal metaplasia.

PATHOLOGICAL STUDIES OF ULCER-CANCER

Pathological studies have dealt with three facets of ulcer-cancers: the chronological relationship between ulcer and cancer; the histogenesis of the cancer; and the histological characteristics of the cancer.

Study of the Chronological Relationship between Ulcer and Cancer

Both Ewing (24) and Mallory (25) have proposed that cancer often becomes ulcerated but that ulcer rarely becomes cancerous. Mallory (25) further postulated that gastric cancer begins as carcinoma in situ (actually intramucosal carcinoma according to current criteria), which then becomes ulcerated, leaving cancer at the margin but not at the base of the ulcer. Strong evidence for the primary nature of the cancer is its location, which is mostly prepyloric, as are gastric cancers in general. The observation of Sakita et al. (11) regarding the life cycle of ulceration and healing of early cancer lends additional support. The realizations that cancer in general, including gastric cancer, has a slow growth rate (26) and that gastric cancer may remain superficial for years (27) make it perfectly reasonable to accept the view that cancer is a primary lesion when it is discovered less than 5 years after the diagnosis of ulcer, albeit the duration of the ulcer before the diagnosis is often unknown.

It is generally accepted that it takes 10 to 15 years for carcinoma to develop in a gastric remnant after partial resection. Yet the average age of patients with ulcer-cancer is in the sixth decade, 50.5 years in one report (8) and 60.7 years in another (18), similar to the average age of patients with gastric ulcer. Among the cases studied by Wenger et al. (12), there was no appreciable age difference between ulcer patients with cancer and those without cancer.

Histogenesis of Ulcer-Cancer

There has been very little information concerning the histogenesis of cancer in a chronic ulcer. Meister et al. (28) noted a high incidence of dysplasia in the ulcerated stomach and a distribution pattern of chronic atrophic gastritis and intestinal metaplasia similar to that in the cancerous stomach. It may be assumed, therefore, that the histogenesis of ulcer-cancer is similar to that of other cancers and is not affected by the ulcer.

Histologic Characteristics of Cancer with Ulcer

Sano (8) noted more cases of signet-ring cell cancers in ulcerated than in nonulcerated early cancers. In a recent report on small and minute early cancers, Hirota et al. (29) noted the ratio of differentiated to undifferentiated cancers was 1:1.8 in ulcerated stomachs and 13.3:1 in nonulcerated stomachs. The undifferentiated cancers included signet-ring cell cancers. A high incidence of infiltrative carcinoma was also noted in advanced ulcerated cancer (30).

EXPERIMENTAL STUDY OF ULCER-CANCER

Experimental studies of ulcer-cancer indicate the preference of cancer development at the ulcer site. Majima et al. (31) embedded beeswax pellets containing 4-nitroquinoline-1-oxide in the gastric wall. The injected site became ulcerated, followed by epithelial proliferation and subsequent cancer. In this experiment it is not surprising that cancer and ulcer were at the same location, since the carcinogen was put at the ulcer site. Takahashi et al. (32) produced ulcer by iodoacetamide in the fundic regions of rat stomach followed by oral administration of N-methyl-N'-nitro-N-nitrosoguanidine. Cancer again developed at the ulcer site. Thus, the chronically ulcerated gastric epithelium appears to be more susceptible to carcinogenic stimulation than the nonulcerated mucosa.

DISCUSSION

There is no question that gastric cancers are often ulcerated and that cancer may develop in a chronic ulcer. While the incidence for the former is rather high, the incidence for the latter is low. The information for early gastric cancer according to Nagayo (10) puts the former at 10 percent and the latter at 0 percent. The latter incidence was based on data for ulcer-cancers.

Ulcer-cancer, defined as the presence of cancer at the margin but not at the base of a chronic ulcer, has often been interpreted as cancer developing in a preexisting chronic ulcer. This interpretation is not necessarily correct in view of the now well-recognized facts that cancer grows slowly and may remain intramucosal for years and that a malignant ulcer can heal. Therefore, an ulcer-cancer may be the result of either cancer developing in an ulcer or the ulceration of a cancer. Conversely, the presence of cancer at the ulcer base does not exclude the possibility of malignant change in the ulcer.

Although pathological features can no longer be relied on for determining whether the cancer has preceded or followed a chronic ulcer, follow-up studies and animal experiments clearly show that a chronic ulcer may become malignant. Experimental studies indicate that the ulcerated gastric epithelium is a favored site for carcinogenic action, possibly because of the immature nature of the regenerating epithelial cells at the ulcer margin. However, the incidence of such an occurrence in humans appears to be low. From the data cited above, the incidence of cancer developing in a chronic ulcer of more than a 5-year duration is around 0.5 to 2 percent, and the incidence of cancer in a stomach resected for clinically benign ulcer is about 2 percent.

More supportive evidence for the malignant transformation of a benign ulcer is the type of cancer seen in ulcer cases. There is a markedly high percentage of signet-ring cell carcinoma as compared with gastric cancer in general. This would not be the case if ulcer occurred randomly on the preexisting cancer. Although benign ulcer often occurs in a metaplastic mucosa, signet-ring cell cancer is not closely associated with metaplasia (see Chapter 12). Thus, the high incidence of this type of cancer cannot be explained on the basis of coincidence.

The development of cancer in ulcer can now be monitored by endoscopic biopsies. Previous follow-up reports showing the discovery of cancer within months to 3 years after the original diagnosis of benignity in nearly one-half of cancer patients (19) indicate a high rate of misdiagnosis. In order to be accurate, multiple biopsies along the ulcer margin are necessary. The procedure clearly has to be guided by the condition of the patient, the size of the ulcer, and complications of the biopsy itself, such as bleeding.

The frequency of misdiagnosis points to the importance of distinguishing a totally benign ulcer from a cancer-harboring one. Of the many differentiating gross features between benign and malignant ulcers, the most important one is the appearance of the mucosa at the ulcer margin. The regenerating marginal mucosa of a benign ulcer is soft, congested, and overhanging, whereas the cancerous tissue is rigid, pale, and sloping toward the ulcer base. Biopsy should be taken from such areas.

REFERENCES

1. Hauser, G. *Das chronische Magengeschwur.* Leipzig: J. B. Hirschfeld, 1883.
2. Hauser, G. *Das cylinderepithel-carcinoma des Magens und des Dickdarms.* Jena: Gusfav. Fischer, 1890.
3. Hauser, G. Die peptische Schadigungen des Magens, des Duodenums und der Speiserohre und der peptische postoperative jejunalgeschwur. In *Handbuch der specizellen pathologischen Anatomic und Histologie,* edited by Henke, F., and Lubarsch, O., pp. 339–811. Berlin: Springer, 1926.
4. Newcomb, W. D. The relationship between peptic ulceration and gastric carcinoma. *Br. J. Surg.* 20 (1933):279–308.
5. Dible, J. H. Gastric ulcer and gastric carcinoma: An inquiry into their relationship. *Br. J. Surg.* 12 (1925):666–700.
6. Oota, K. Role of gastric ulcer in the causation of gastric cancer in Japan: A histopathological study of 3,000 gastrectomy materials. *Acta Un. Int. Cancer* 19 (1963):1208–1209.
7. Kuru, M. *Atlas of Early Carcinoma of the Stomach.* Tokyo: Nakayama-Shoten, 1967.
8. Sano, R. Pathological analysis of 300 cases of early gastric cancer with special reference to cancer associated with ulcer. *Gann Monogr. Cancer Res.* 11 (1971):81–89.
9. Oota, K. Early phases of development of human gastric cancer. *Gann Monogr. Cancer Res.* 18 (1976):77–83.
10. Nagayo, T. Precursors of human gastric cancer: Their frequencies and histological characteristics. In *Pathophysiology of Carcinogenesis in Digestive Organs,* edited by Farber, E., Kawachi, T., Nagayo, T., Sugano, H., Sugimura, T., and Weisburger, J. H., pp. 151–161. Tokyo: University of Tokyo Press, 1977.
11. Sakita, T., Oguro, Y., Takasu, S., Fukutomi, H., Miwa, T., and Yoshimori, M. Observations on the healing of ulcerations in early gastric cancer; the life cycle of the malignant ulcer. *Gastroenterology* 60 (1971):835–844.
12. Wenger, J., Brandborg, L. L., and Spellman, F. A. The Veterans Administration cooperative study on gastric ulcer. 6. Cancer. *Gastroenterology* 61 (1971):598–605.
13. Majima, S., Yamaguchi, I., Teshima, T., and Karube, K. On malignant change of gastric ulcer. *Tohoku J. Exp. Med.* 86 (1965):255–276.
14. Ihre, B. J. E., Barr, H., and Havermark, G. Ulcer cancer of the stomach—A follow up study of 473 cases of gastric ulcer. *Gastroenterologia* 102 (1964):78–91.
15. Yamagata, S., and Hisamichi, S. Precancerous lesions of the stomach. *World J. Surg.* 3 (1979):671–673.
16. Haukland, H. H., Johnson, J. A., and Eide, J. T. Carcinoma diagnosed in excised gastric ulcers. *Acta Chir. Scand.* 147 (1981):439–443.
17. Hirohata, T. Mortality from gastric cancer and other causes after medical or surgical treatment of gastric ulcer. *J. Natl. Cancer Inst.* 41 (1968):895–908.
18. Larson, N. E., Cain, J. C., and Bartholomew, L. G. Prognosis of the medically treated small gastric ulcer, II. Ten years follow-up study of 391 patients. *N. Engl. J. Med.* 264 (1961):330–334.

19. Thunold, S., and Wetteland, P. Ulcer carcinoma of the stomach in a 10-year biopsy series. A follow-up study of 19 patients. *Acta Pathol. Microbiol. Scand.* 56 (1962):155–165.
20. Kawai, K., Kizu, M., and Miyaoka, T. Epidemiology and pathogenesis of gastric cancer. *Front. Gastrointest. Res.* 6 (1980):71–86.
21. Montgomery, R. D., and Richardson, B. P. Gastric ulcer and cancer. *Q. J. Med.* 44 (1975):591–599.
22. Swynnerton, B. F., and Tanner, N. C. Chronic gastric ulcer. A comparison between a gastroscopically controlled series treated medically and a series treated by surgery. *Br. Med. J.* 2 (1953):841–847.
23. Stemmermann, G., Haenszel, W., and Locke, F. Epidemiologic pathology of gastric ulcer and gastric carcinoma among Japanese in Hawaii. *J. Natl. Cancer Inst.* 58 (1977):13–20.
24. Ewing, J. *Neoplastic Diseases*, 4th ed., pp. 689–695. Philadelphia: W. B. Saunders, 1940.
25. Mallory, T. B. Carcinoma in situ of the stomach and its bearing on the histogenesis of malignant ulcers. *Arch. Pathol.* 30 (1940):348–362.
26. Clarkson, B., Ota, T., Okhita, T., and O'Conner, A. Kinetics of proliferation of cancer cells in neoplastic effusions in man. *Cancer* 18 (1965):1189–1213.
27. Fugita, S., and Hattori, T. Cell proliferation, differentiation and migration in the gastric mucosa. A study on the background of carcinogenesis. In *Pathophysiology of Carcinogenesis in Digestive Organs*, edited by Farber, E., Kawachi, T., Nagayo, T., Sugano, H., Sugimura, T., and Weisburger, J. H., pp. 21–36. Tokyo: University of Tokyo Press, 1977.
28. Meister, H., Holubarsch, Ch., Haferkamp, O., Schlag, P., and Herfarth, Ch. Gastritis, intestinal metaplasia and dysplasia versus benign ulcer in stomach and duodenum and gastric carcinoma. A histotopographical study. *Pathol. Res. Pract.* 164 (1979):259–269.
29. Hirota, T., Itabashi, M., Suzuki, K., and Yoshida, S. Clinicopathologic study of minute and small early gastric cancer. Histogenesis of gastric cancer. *Pathol. Annu.* 15 (1980):1–19.
30. Ming, S.-C. Gastric carcinoma. A pathobiological classification. *Cancer* 39 (1977):2475–2485.
31. Majima, S., Takahashi, T., Yoshida, K., Karube, K., Machida, T., Narisama, T., Hoshi, H., Hiroki, T., Ito, K., and Kurata, Y. Atypical epithelial proliferation in the course of experimental production of ulcer-carcinoma of the stomach. *Tohoku J. Exp. Med.* 93 (1967):363–376.
32. Takahashi, M., Shirai, T., Gukushima, S., Hahanouchi, M., and Hirose, M. Effects of fundic ulcers induced by iodoacetamide on development of gastric tumors in rats treated with N-methyl-N'-nitro-N-nitrosoguanidine. *Gann* 67 (1976):47–54.

22 POSSIBLE CORRELATION BETWEEN STOMACH ULCER AND CANCER

A. Bajtai and J. Juhász

FREQUENCY AND PATHOLOGY: REVIEW OF THE LITERATURE

In 1829 Cruveilhier (1) presented the hypothesis that cancer might develop at the site of a gastric ulcer. In 1842 Rokitansky (2) and in 1859 Brinton (3) confirmed this supposition. Since then, the existence, frequency, clinical picture, and morphological substrate of carcinoma have been vividly discussed. The intensity of the dispute has not subsided after 150 years of discussion.

There has been evidence of an undeniable correlation between ulcer and cancer, in some cases at least. The pessimistic opinion of Ewing (4) that this correlation was rather remote has not been unequivocally upheld. Although the existence of ulcer-carcinoma cannot be denied since the study of Hauser (5), its frequency and morphological substrate as well as its early diagnosis have raised many questions. The frequency rate has been decreasing to some extent since the turn of the century when Wilson and McCarty (6) estimated it at 71 percent. It is to be remarked that such high rates are often based upon surgical observations, not infrequently without histological confirmation. According to the data of Fischer (7), the acceptable frequency varies between 1 and 20 percent in the English and American literature up to 1941. In 1959 Robbins (8) estimated this rate at 1 percent only. In 1962 Stevenson (9) spoke of 2 to 3 percent.

Marshall and Adamson (10) rejected the precancerous character of gastric ulcer. Ackerman and Del Regato (11) believed that an extremely small number of gastric ulcers can undergo carcinomatous changes.

According to Robbins (8), the ratio of benign to malignant ulcers was 3:1, independent of age. Fifty-six percent of malignant and 58 percent of benign ulcers were localized in the pyloric canal. Between 1935 and 1964 Becker and Mayland (12) examined the data from 1,875 patients with gastric cancer and those from 1,545 patients with ulcer. They observed 60 cases of ulcer carcinoma, representing a frequency of 3.1 percent among the gastric cancers and 3.7 percent among the ulcers. They (12) also observed ulcer-carcinoma in 15 percent of operated stomachs. According to them, the actual frequency rate lay around 10 percent, but at the time of the operation, the advanced state of the tumors did not allow the observation of the signs of antecedent peptic ulcer described by Newcomb (13) and Askanazy (14). The difference in the frequencies of ulcer-carcinoma could be attributed partly to geographic fluctuations of ulcer and cancer and partly to the different methods of evaluation.

The location, shape, and size of the ulcer undergoing carcinomatous transformation have no characteristics. Alvarez and McCarty (15) found that ulcers exceeding 1.5 centimeters are suspicious for malignant transformation. Comfort and Butsch (16) believed that ulcers larger than 4.5 centimeters most probably degenerate into malignancy. These opinions cannot be maintained anymore. According to Robbins (8) 10 percent of ulcers exceeding 4 centimeters were benign, whereas 20 percent of those smaller than 2 centimeters were malignant. The latter ones were particularly capable of early metastasis.

In 1971 Sano (17) in Japan studied 300 early gastric cancers. Of his material 211 (70.3 percent) were associated with peptic ulcer. He also pointed out that in the early phase of ulcer-cancer, the cancer was in the marginal part of the ulcer. The histogenesis of ulcer-cancer was regarded as due to cancerization of regenerating epithelium in the marginal mucosa of the peptic ulcer. This epithelium became erosive whenever the ulcer was active. Moreover, in the surrounding tissue there was multifocal, ofttimes severe atrophic gastritis. These chronic stimuli led to alternating destruction and regeneration of the gastric epithelium. The malignant transformation might be considered a result of the aforementioned processes.

According to Sano (17) the early gastric carcinomas associated with chronic peptic ulcer were localized in the area of the gastric angle. Other early carcinomas, frequently the protruded types, could be found in the pyloric region. In the latter area, intestinal metaplasia was very frequent. The carcinomas associated with chronic ulcer were signet-ring cell or undifferentiated tumors. The early cancers without peptic ulcer were differentiated adenocarcinomas. Sano (17) found a difference in the age distribution and mean age. Cancer with concomitant ulcer was more prevalent among younger people.

Some investigators attributed a better prognosis to ulcer-cancer compared with other types of gastric carcinoma (17–19). However, the disturbance of local lymphatic circulation in the ulcerated area (20) might promote an early dissemination of the tumor cells, and the histological type of these tumors (signet-ring cell carcinoma) is known to have a very poor prognosis.

According to Gebhardt et al. (18), a local resection of the stomach was sufficient for the treatment of an ulcer-cancer, depending on the location and size of the tumor. Their good results after such a resection, the 5-year survival rates being 100 percent for the early carcinomas and 67.7 percent for other tumors, indicated that a total gastrectomy for the ulcer-cancer was unnecessary.

Rényi-Vámos and Szinay (20) demonstrated a severe disturbance of local lymphatic circulation in the deep layers and surroundings of penetrating and scarring peptic ulcers. Therefore, early spread and dissemination of a small cancer could develop in the macroscopically normal gastric mucosa.

The lymphatic vessels at the junction of the mucosa and submucosa are frequently dilated. Early invasion of cancer could be found very often at this point. In many tissue blocks cut from the surroundings of ulcer-cancers, we have found that carcinoma could extend below the macroscopically normal mucosa for a great distance. In this way tumor cell emboli could grow into the normal gastric mucosa, as shown in Figures 22-1 to 22-3, in which the lymphatic vessels over and under the muscularis mucosae were filled with tumor cells.

The significance of local lymphatic circulation must be emphasized in the early forms of ulcer-cancer. The cancer in these cases is located in the marginal mucosa surrounding the ulcer. While there is not yet any sign of carcinomatous invasion into the deeper layers of the stomach wall, the cancer cells may spread along the gastric wall and invade the dilated lymphatic vessels. In this way the lymphatic outflow produces metastasis in the regional lymph nodes. This sequence of events was illustrated by one of our patients, a 21-year-old male, whose ulcer-cancer is shown in Figure 22-4. The tumor was

(Text continues on page 278)

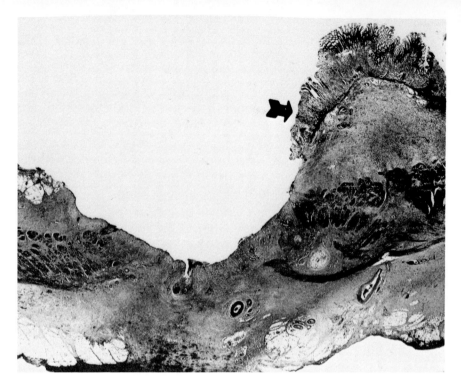

Figure 22-1.　Survey picture of a characteristic chronic ulcer. In the middle, note the dense scar tissue disrupting the layer of muscularis propria. Cancer developed at the edge of the ulcer (*arrow*). H&E stain. × 1.5.

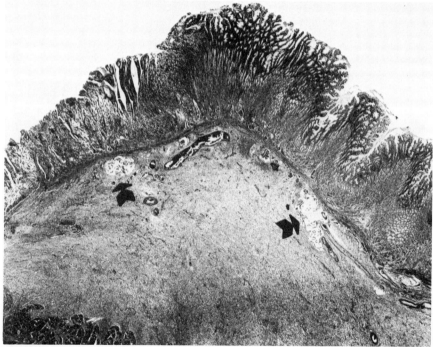

Figure 22-2.　The margin of the ulcer shown in Figure 22-1. Note the tumorous transformation of the mucosa on the left. The lymph vessels under the muscularis mucosae were filled with cancer cell emboli (*arrows*). H&E stain. × 40.

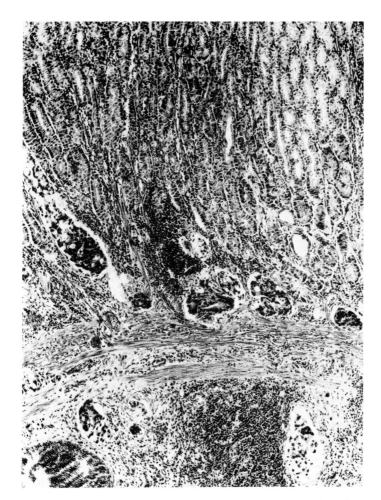

Figure 22-3.   The same case as shown in Figure 22-1. Retrograde lymphatic infiltration of the gastric mucosa by tumor cell emboli. H&E stain. × 160.

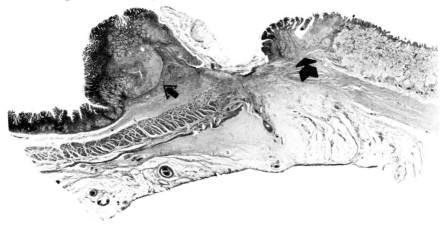

Figure 22-4.   An excavated prepyloric lesion of a 21-year-old male. In the middle is the tumorfree chronic ulcer. Malignant transformation was present only in the marginal mucosa (*arrows*). On the left note the tumor invasion into the submucosa. There was no infiltration in the deeper layer. H&E stain. × 1.5.

confined to the mucosa. There was no sign of carcinomatous invasion into the deeper layers of the gastric wall. The follow-up of the patient later showed the early dissemination of cancer cells by lymph vessels. The tumor was histologically a signet-ring cell carcinoma.

Gebhardt et al. (18) assumed the view that the tumors that had partially infiltrated the ulcer floor were not ulcer-cancers, but rather were primary carcinomas with secondary ulceration. It is possible that a peptic ulceration might develop in a tumor if some gastric acid secretion is present. But how could it occur in an anacid patient?

In the initial stage, the features described by Hauser (5), Askanazy (14), and Newcomb (13) can be readily recognized: The tumor-free part of the excavated lesion must show the characteristic features of a chronic peptic ulcer (Figure 22-5). In the advanced phase (Figures 22-6 and 22-7), the tumor cells infiltrate the base of excavated lesion and the aforesaid features may no longer be evident. For the most part, only such indirect evidence as obliterating endangiitis or irregular growth of nerve fibers (amputation neurinomas) in the surrounding tissue indicates the presence of a preexisting ulcer. In the final stage (Figure 22-8), all the surface area of the excavated lesion is infiltrated by tumorous tissue. Only the dense scar tissue, permeating and disrupting the muscularis propria, can hint at the true nature of the process.

Sakita et al. (21) have observed significant healing in 70 percent of 72 malignant ulcers found in a group of 122 cases of early gastric cancer. A careful follow-up of a 50-year-old female revealed a cycle of healing and recurrence of ulceration in a malignant stomach ulcer. The "life cycle" theory based on this finding is very interesting, but it is convincing only if step-sectioning biopsy is performed in every phase of the patient's follow-up. The latter point must be emphasized because of the long-lasting development of carcinomatous growth within the stomach mucosa.

It is well known from the cytological investigations of Loux and Zamcheck (22) that the period of time from the first positive cytological finding to the first macroscopical change in the stomach mucosa takes at least 5 years. Fujita and Hattori (23) put the period of time from the onset of the early carcinoma to clinical manifestation at 16 to 17 years. In such a long-lasting process, the development of a recurrent ulcer is possible.

It is a very great problem to identify the origin of an ulcer-cancer. Kawai et al. (24), observing 408 follow-up cases of chronic peptic ulcer for more than 6 months, found 4 ulcer-cancers. One of them showed the possibility of malignant transformation in a benign ulcer scar. At times, however, an ulcer scar with irregular folds cannot be

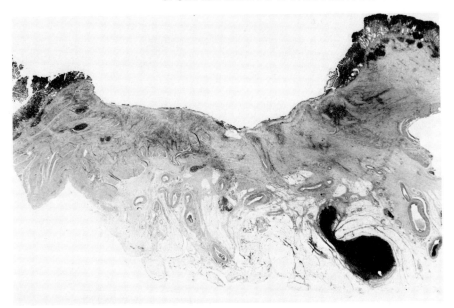

Figure 22-5.   Typical early ulcer-cancer. The excavation was 4 centimeters in diameter. The base of the ulcer contained only dense scar tissue and adipose tissue of the great omentum. Superficial carcinomatous infiltration was present in the marginal zone of the ulcer. H&E stain. × 1.5.

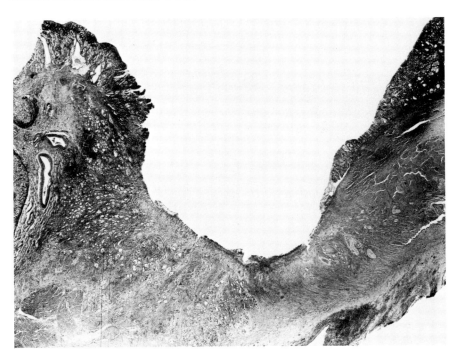

Figure 22-6.   Deep excavation of an ulcer-cancer partly infiltrated by carcinomatous tissue in the base of the ulcer. H&E stain. × 2.

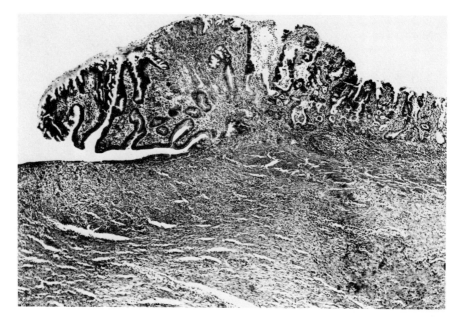

Figure 22-7.   The same case as shown in Figure 22-6. Proliferation of malignant glands at the edge of the ulcer. H&E stain. × 80.

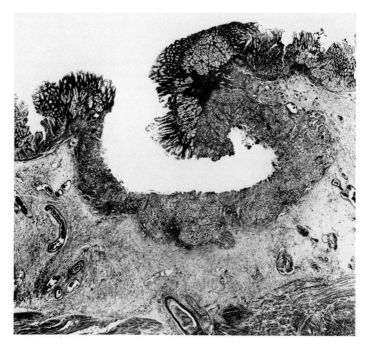

Figure 22-8.   The entire surface area of the excavated lesion was infiltrated by tumorous tissue. There is no sign of peptic ulceration. H&E stain. × 1.5.

reliably differentiated from a gastric carcinoma, and therefore endoscopy with biopsy may be required (25).

The morphology of the blood vessels in and around a peptic ulcer has been dealt with by many investigators. Arteriosclerosis leading to significant narrowing or complete obstruction of the vessels supplying the stomach is infrequent. There is apparently no relationship between arteriosclerosis and vascular changes in association with a cicatrized peptic ulcer. The inflammatory process progressing from the ulceration to the vascular wall can involve arteries as well as veins.

Juhász (26) has studied the vascular changes in 51 ulcer-cancers in a group of 443 surgically removed gastric carcinomas. It was observed that in arteries lying under the serosa and in the scar replacing the destroyed muscular layer of the stomach, an intimal hyperplasia could be seen. The arteries contain a remarkably large amount of elastic fibers arranged either concentrically or occasionally eccentrically. This change is sharply demarcated from the intimal proliferation in vessels running immediately under the ulcer surface. In the latter a necrotizing panarteritis and consequent occlusion can be found. They result occasionally in thrombosis. The regenerating epithelium at the ulcer edge requires an adequate vascular supply. It is tempting to speculate that a decrease in this supply together with continuous mechanical and chemical irritation may possibly lead to abnormal epithelial regeneration.

OUR MATERIALS

A total of 433 surgically resected stomach cancers was recorded and verified histologically. Of them 89 (20.5 percent) were associated with chronic peptic ulcer. This was much less than reported by Sano (17), who found an ulcer and cancer association in 70 percent of early gastric cancers.

Our cases included 88 early gastric cancers (20.3 percent of all carcinomas). Among them 44 cases, one-half of all the early stomach carcinomas, showed an association with chronic peptic ulcer.

In the remaining 345 cases of advanced gastric cancer, the tumor was associated with chronic ulcer in 45 cases (13 percent).

The peak incidence in both types of tumor was in the seventh decade. The male-to-female ratio was 2:1. The early cancers were located in both the prepyloric region along the lesser curvature and the gastric angle region. There was no difference among these findings between the cancers with and without peptic ulcer.

We have not found a correlation between the size and shape of chronic ulcer and its malignant transformation. On one hand, a large, several times recurrent peptic ulcer turned out to be benign at the time of surgical intervention. On the other, carcinoma developed in the surroundings of a peptic ulcer 10 to 15 millimeters in diameter. The lack of correlation between the size of the ulcer and cancer development was illustrated by two cases, both of which had a large, penetrating ulcer and a small ulcer in the stomach. Early cancer was found in the small ulcers, one of which was scarred, and not in the large ulcer. In another case of healing peptic ulcer, early malignant transformation developed in the linear scarring part of the lesion, whereas the fibrinoid necrotic area was free of tumor.

Chronic ulcer and atrophic gastritis are both precancerous conditions (27). These two diseases frequently occur together. Stadelmann and Miederer (28) pointed out that the higher the ulcer is in the stomach, the more extensive and severe will be the gastritis. In the step-sectioning of biopsy materials obtained from patients suffering from chronic peptic ulcer, we have found severe atrophic gastritis around the ulcer in 43 percent of patients.

CONCLUSIONS

The malignant transformation of benign gastric ulcer is indisputable, but its frequency is still uncertain. The location of ulcer suspicious of carcinomatous change is not characteristic, and neither is the shape nor size of the ulcer.

Ulcer-cancer is an early carcinoma in which the ulceration extends beyond the muscularis mucosae or there is a massive scar tissue extending to the serosa at the base of the ulcer. Since cicatrization splits the muscularis mucosae and the muscularis propria, the fusion of the two muscular layers can be observed at the margin of the ulcer, and obliterant endangiitis as well as amputation neurinomas may be present.

Tumor cannot be regarded as ulcer-cancer if the base of the ulcer shows a tumorous infiltration or if its margins are free of tumor and the morphological signs indicating chronic ulcer are missing.

It has to be kept in mind that tumorous proliferation may develop not only on the margin of an ulcer, but also in the scar of a healed ulcer. On the other hand, chronic atrophic gastritis with severe dysplasia is not infrequent around an ulcer or in an ulcer scar. The latter should not be confused with cancer.

The step-sectioning of biopsy material has particular importance not only in the diagnosis but in the follow-up of patients suffering from gastric ulcer. Multiple biopsy from different points around the ulcer must be repeated during the follow-up, so as to prove the true nature of the ulcerative process in the stomach.

REFERENCES

1. Cruveilhier, J. *Anatomie pathologique de corps humain, Vol. 1*, pp. 1829–1835. Paris: J. B. Bailliére, 1829.
2. Rokitansky, C., von. *Handbuch der speziellen pathologischen Anatomie*. Wien: W. Braumüller, 1842.
3. Brinton, W. *The diseases of the Stomach with an Introduction on its Anatomy and Physiology*. London: John Churchill, 1859.
4. Ewing, J. The beginnings of gastric cancer. *Am. J. Surg.* 31 (1936):204–206.
5. Hauser, G. *Das chronische Magengeschwür*. Leipzig: J. B. Hirschfeld, 1883.
6. Wilson, L. B., and McCarty, W. C. Pathological relationship of gastric ulcer and gastric carcinoma. *Am. J. Med. Sci.* 138 (1909):846–853.
7. Fischer, W. Einiges über Magengeschwür, Magenkrebs und ihre Beziehungen zueinander. *Med. Klin.* 37 (1941):4–7.
8. Robbins, S. L. Contributions of the pathologist to presentday concepts of gastric ulcer. *JAMA* 171 (1959):2053–2055.
9. Stevenson, J. K. Gastric carcinoma. In *Surgery of Stomach and Duodenum*, edited by Harkins, H. N., and Nyhus, L. M., pp. 352–387. Boston: Little, Brown, 1962.
10. Marshall, S. F., and Adamson, N. E. Cancer of the stomach: Follow-up study of 1708 patients. *South. Med. J.* 50 (1957):776–783.
11. Ackerman, L. V., and Del Regato, J. A. *Cancer Diagnosis, Treatment and Prognosis*, 4th ed., p. 430. St. Louis: C. V. Mosby, 1970.
12. Becker, Th., and Mayland, J. Das Ulcuskarzinom des Magens. *Zbl. Chir.* 91 (1966):68–75.
13. Newcomb, W. D. The relationship between peptic ulceration and gastric carcinoma. *Br. J. Surg.* 220 (1933):279–308.
14. Askanazy, M. Über Bau und Entstehung des chronischen Magengeschwürs sowie Soorpilzbefunde in ihm. *Virchows Arch. (Pathol. Anat.)* 250 (1924):370–486.
15. Alvarez, W. C., and McCarty, W. C. Size of resected gastric ulcers and gastric carcinomas. *JAMA* 91 (1928):226–231.
16. Comfort, M. W., and Butsch, W. J. Gastric acidity in cases of benign and malignant small lesions of the stomach. *Proc. Mayo Clin.* 11 (1936):440–446.
17. Sano, R. Pathological analysis of 300 cases of early gastric cancer. With special reference to cancer associated with ulcers. *Gann Monogr. Cancer Res.* 11 (1971):81–89.
18. Gebhardt, Ch., Moschinski, D., Hoffmann, E., and Gebhardt, G. Das Ulcuscarcinom des Magens. *Langenbecks Arch. Chir.* 343 (1977):113–122.
19. Haukland, H. H., Johnson, J. A., and Eide, J. T. Carcinoma diagnosed in excised gastric ulcers. *Acta Chir. Scand.* 147 (1981):439–443.

20. Rényi-Vámos, F., and Szinay, G. Y. Das Lymphgefässsystem des Magens und sein Verhalten bei Ulcus Ventriculi. *Acta Morphol. Acad. Sci. Hung.* 4 (1954): 353–365.

21. Sakita, T., Oguro, Y., Takasu, S., Fukutomi, H., Miwa, T., and Yoshimori, M. Observations on the healing of ulcerations in early gastric cancer. The life cycle of the malignant ulcer. *Gastroenterology* 60 (1971):835–844.

22. Loux, H. A., and Zamcheck, N. Cytological evidence for the long "quiescent" stage of gastric cancer in 2 patients with pernicious anemia. *Gastroenterology* 57 (1969):173–184.

23. Fujita, S., and Hattori, T. Cell proliferation, differentiation and migration in the gastric mucosa. A study on the background carcinogenesis. In *Pathophysiology of Carcinogenesis in Digestive Organs*, edited by Farber, E., Kawachi, T., Nagayo, T., Sugano, H., Sugimura, T., and Weisburger, J. H., pp. 21–36. Tokyo: University of Tokyo Press, 1977.

24. Kawai, K., Akasaka, Y., and Kohli, Y. Endoscopical approach to the "malignant change of benign gastric ulcer" from our follow-up studies. *Endoscopy* 5 (1973):53–60.

25. Gelfand, D. W., and Ott, D. J. Gastric ulcer scars. *Radiology* 140 (1981):37–43.

26. Juhász, J. The role of vascular lesions in the malignant transformation of chronic peptic ulcer. *Acta Morphol. Acad. Sci. Hung.* 16 (1968):41–52.

27. Grundmann, E., and Schlake, W. Histology of possible precancerous stages in the stomach. In *Gastric Cancer*, edited by Herfarth, Ch., and Schlag, P., pp. 72–82. Berlin: Springer-Verlag, 1979.

28. Stadelmann, O., and Miederer, S. E. Die umschriebenen Schleimhautveränderungen des Magens—ein differentialdiagnostisches und klinisches Problem. *Schweiz. Rundschau. Med.* 60 (1971):1358–1364.

VII POSTRESECTION GASTRIC STUMP

23 CARCINOMA OF THE RESECTED STOMACH

A. Gad

Sixty years after the initial description of carcinoma of the resected stomach (1), many questions remain unanswered about the
nature of this development, its pathogenesis, and frequency. Disagreement exists as to whether the possible causal relationship is attribut-
able to the gastrectomy procedure itself or to the underlying gastric
pathology or to both of these.

Several contradictory reports about the incidence of this condition have been published by European and Scandinavian authors. Earlier reports were based on clinical and autopsy studies (2–14). With
the introduction of fiber endoscopy, however, adequate follow-up
has been made possible and prospective studies have been carried out
(15–20). Most interest has been focused on Billroth II (B-II)-operated
patients, but carcinoma developing after Billroth I (B-I) gastrectomy,
gastroenterostomy, and vagotomy with or without pyloroplasty has
been the subject of sporadic reports (21–25).

The main concern of this chapter is to investigate the sequelae of
B-II gastrectomy for benign disease, with special emphasis on the like-
lihood of organizing follow-up schemes of gastrectomized patients.

Such schemes should be seriously considered if convincing evidence is provided that these patients are at a sufficiently high risk for developing carcinoma in the resected stomach.

MATERIALS AND METHODS

The number of inhabitants of Kopparberg County, situated in the middle of Sweden, has been fairly stable during the last decade. In 1977 the mean population was 285,018 and was nearly equally divided between males and females.

The material of this investigation was based on 2,723 patients who, according to the operation register, underwent B-II partial gastrectomy for benign conditions from 1909 to 1973 in the four main hospitals of the county, namely, Falun, Mora, Ludvika, and Avesta, as detailed in Table 23-1.

The operation was performed for gastric ulcer in 22.8 percent, duodenal ulcer in 47.0 percent, simultaneous gastric and duodenal ulcers in 2.2 percent, and gastroduodenal ulcer not otherwise specified in 27.7 percent. Gastritis was the cause of operation in only seven patients (0.3 percent) during the whole period.

Until late 1957 antecolic anastomosis without enteroanastomosis was the standard procedure in the four main hospitals. Enteroanastomosis was performed in one-half of the patients who underwent B-II gastrectomy at Falun Hospital from September 1957 to September 1959, and became routine after September 1959 (26).

Table 23-1. The Distribution of Billroth II Gastrectomy Patients according to the Cause of Operation and Operative Mortality in Kopparberg County, Sweden, between 1909 and 1973

	Cause of Operation						
Period	Gastritis	Gastric Ulcer	Duodenal Ulcer	Gastro-duodenal Ulcer	Gastro-duodenal Ulcer not Otherwise Specified	Operative Mortality	Total
1909–40	—	96	75	24	45	18	240
1941–46 (Estimate)	—	15	41	13	87	10	156
1947–55	2	69	166	10	402	29	649
1956–64	2	337	722	14	160	40	1,235
1965–73	3	105	276	—	59	11	443
Total	7	622	1,280	61	753	108	2,723
%	0.3	22.8	47.0	2.2	27.7	4.0	100.0

Operative mortality during the 65 years occurred in 108 patients (4 percent), and the remaining 2,615 were the target of this long-term investigation, the ultimate aim of which was to trace as many of these patients as possible. This was to be achieved partly retrospectively by examining autopsy records and death certificates and partly prospectively by the organized or nonorganized follow-up activities taking place in the four main hospitals of the county. In 1976 patients operated on at Falun Hospital from September 1957 to September 1959 were invited to follow-up by the Department of Gastroenterology. The 237 patients in this group were included in a randomized study of the afferent loop syndrome after B-II gastrectomy with antecolic gastroenterostomy with and without enteroanastomosis (26). The nonorganized follow-up included symptomatic gastrectomized patients who sought medical advice for gastrointestinal or other troubles.

The follow-up comprised a detailed history, physical examination, necessary laboratory investigations, upper gastrointestinal X-ray film when indicated, and gastroscopy. During gastroscopy multiple brushings for cytology and biopsy specimens for histology were routinely taken. The standard biopsy sites were the afferent and efferent loops, stoma, posterior wall, and random parts of the rest of the gastric remnant. Additional specimens were taken from lesions discovered at gastroscopy, and the total number of biopsies ranged between 5 and 12 per patient. According to the original plan, the follow-up was to be performed annually.

Until the end of June 1983, a total of 292 patients was traced. They belonged to one of three groups as shown in Table 23-2. Forty-six patients did not receive any follow-up, but were entered in the study after the discovery of carcinoma in the resected stomach (18 cases) or the diagnosis of or death from other disease conditions (28 cases). Nineteen patients were followed up by physical examination and endoscopy, whereas 227 were fully followed up according to the prospective scheme, more than one-third of them being subjected to two to seven examinations.

The patients, 233 males and 59 females (4:1 ratio), were operated on according to B-II-type partial gastrectomy for benign disease from 1927 to 1973 (Figure 23-1). All patients were operated on in Kopparberg County except nine who were operated on in other parts of Sweden, namely, Stockholm (three), Gävle (two), Karlstad (two), Västerås (one), and Kiruna (one). Available records as well as all histology and cytology slides were reviewed.

Slides from the gastrectomy specimen of a patient originally considered to have had a benign duodenal ulcer were found on review to

Table 23-2. The Distribution of 292 Patients according
to Type of Follow-Up

| | Type of Follow-Up | | | |
	Physical Examination, Endoscopy, Cytology, and Biopsy	Physical Examination and Endoscopy	No Follow-Up	Total
No. of patients	227[a]	19[b]	46[c]	292
No. of cancer cases	5	—	18	23
No. of deaths	19	3	33	55

[a]Five patients operated on outside Kopparberg County; none developed cancer.
[b]One patient operated on outside Kopparberg County; no cancer.
[c]Three patients operated on outside Kopparberg County; all developed cancer.

contain small groups of Grimelius-positive carcinoid tumor cells in the fibrous tissue of the ulcer base. This patient developed liver and lung metastases 13 years after operation and was excluded from the study. A patient considered to have had intramucosal gastric carcinoma was included in this study as no carcinoma was seen on review of the original slides, which showed only hyperplasia of the glandular epithelium bordering a benign peptic ulcer. This case was found during the review of gastric cancers recorded in the files of our department from 1965 to 1978.

The nature of the benign disease resulting in operation could not be identified in 44.6 percent of the cases, and the type of ulcer, whether gastric or duodenal, was not specified in 23.3 percent. Duodenal and gastric ulcers had an equal share of 14.7 percent each. Coexistent gastric and duodenal ulcers were present in 1.7 percent. Gastritis was the sole underlying cause of operation in 1 percent only. The age at operation ranged from 17 to 79 years, with an average of 43.5 years, as detailed in Figure 23-2. The follow-up period was counted as the time lapsed between the date of the operation and the date of the latest follow-up or death for every individual patient. It ranged from 5 to 50 years with an average of 21.2 years, 82 percent of the patients being followed-up for 11 to 30 years, as illustrated in Figure 23-3. A total of 48 patients died during the period of study because of carcinoma developing in the gastric remnant and other malignant or nonmalignant diseases. Carcinoma of the urinary bladder, breast, pros-

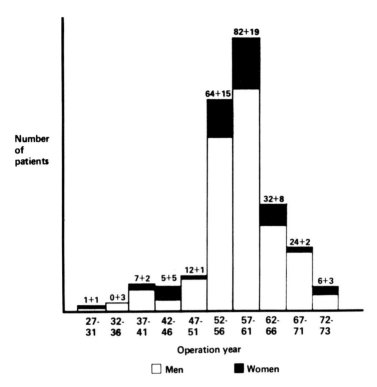

Figure 23-1.   The number of patients operated on at 5-year intervals between 1927 and 1973.

tate, larynx, and lung and malignant melanoma were diagnosed in a number of survivals.

All biopsies and resection specimens were fixed in 10 percent formalin and processed in the usual manner. New sections were cut during the review when necessary and stained with special procedures such as alcian blue (pH 2.5)/periodic acid-Schiff and high-iron diamine/alcian blue for the characterization of epithelial mucosubstances, the Gordon and Sweet silver impregnation method for reticular fibers, and the Grimelius method for argyrophilic cells. On histopathological examination the presence of gastritis, intestinal metaplasia, lipid islands, cystically dilated glands, erosions, ulcers, polyps, and dysplasia was especially noted. Dysplasia was classified into mild, moderate, and severe, using criteria based on those described by Nagayo (27).

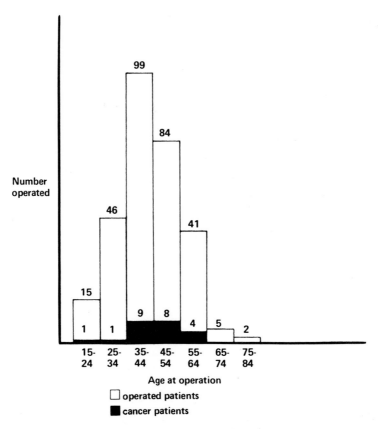

Figure 23-2.   The distribution of patients according to age at operation and the number of cancer cases in each age group.

RESULTS

No information was available concerning the symptoms and signs in a group of 63 patients (21.6 percent). Only 27 patients (9.2 percent)

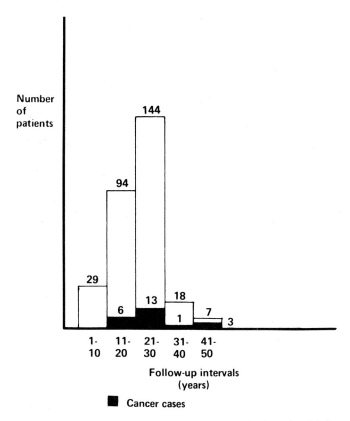

Figure 23-3. The distribution of patients according to the length of follow-up and the number of cancer cases in each period.

were symptomfree since the operation was performed, but the majority presented with a wide range of complaints, often more than one at the same time, the most frequent association being pain, bleeding, and anemia. The common symptoms and signs were diffuse or epigastric pain (31.4 percent), anemia (22.3 percent), ulcer-type dyspepsia (16.6 percent), nausea and/or vomiting (16.2 percent), bleeding (16.2 percent) in the form of hematemesis, melena, or both, and weight loss (14.0 percent). Dumping syndrome, anorexia, and diarrhea were reported in a few cases.

Endoscopic findings were lacking in 50 cases (17.1 percent) either because endoscopy was not performed or because the results of the examination were not available. The gastric remnant was endo-scopically normal in 15 persons (6.2 percent) only. The most common endoscopic finding was gastritis, one or the other type of which was reported in 64.5 percent of the patients either alone or together with other findings such as bile regurgitation (21.5 percent), polyps and pseudopolyps (16.5 percent), ulcers (14.5 percent), and lipid islands (11.2 percent). Ulcers were often stomal and were the main cause of bleeding when present. Fungus infection was thought to be present in 15 cases (5.5 percent), but its presence was histologically confirmed in 5 cases only. Leukoplakia, hiatal hernia, intestinal metaplasia, and reflux esophagitis were reported in a minority of cases.

Histologic and/or cytologic results were available in 227 patients and were normal in 17.1 percent. Different types of gastritis with or without intestinal metaplasia, cystically dilated glands, surface epithe-lial papillary or villous formations, and lipid islands were reported in 55.7 percent. Ulcers and polyps, hyperplastic or adenovillous, had an equal frequency of 5.7 percent each. Dysplasia was initially diagnosed in 56 (24.7 percent) of the patients who were prospectively followed up (Table 23-3). Inflammation associated with slight dysplasia was the predominant type (71.4 percent), and follow-up so far has revealed that most of the dysplasias regressed. Progression from slight to mod-erate dysplasia took place in two patients after 2 years and stump car-cinoma developed in the third (case no. 17 in Table 23-4) 17 months after the report of slight dysplasia in the biopsy material. However, 25 (44.6 percent) of the patients with dysplasia were lost to follow-up.

Altogether, 23 B-II-operated patients developed cancer in the re-sected stomach. Table 23-4 summarizes the relevant clinical, patholo-gic, and follow-up data of these cases. The patients, 18 males and 5

Table 23-3. The Degree and Fate of Dysplasia in 56 Cases of the Prospective Study Group

Dysplasia			Fate		
Degree	No. of Patients	Lost to Follow-Up	Stationary	Regression	Progression
Slight	40	15	3	19	3
Moderate	13	8	1	4	—
Severe	3	2	—	1	—
Total	56	25	4	24	3

females (3.6:1 ratio), ranged in age from 24 to 62 years at the time of operation, with an average of 45.4 years. The number of cancers developing in patients in different age groups at the time of operation is illustrated in Figure 23-2. The initial disease was gastric ulcer in 12 patients, duodenal ulcer in 9, and both in 2. Gastroenterostomy was antecolic in 18 patients and retrocolic in 5, and enteroanastomosis was performed as a part of the operation in 2 cases and 12 years later in 1 case. All patients were operated on for the initial disease in Kopparberg County except for patient nos. 3, 7, and 18 (Table 23-4) who were operated on in Gävle, Stockholm, and Karlstad, respectively. At the time of cancer diagnosis, the age of the patients ranged from 59 to 88 years, with an average of 71.6 years. Family history of gastric carcinoma was positive in one patient whose mother died with the same disease.

All cancers were diagnosed between 1967 and 1983, 14 of them between 1969 and 1979. These 14 cancers constituted 1.9 percent of 756 gastric cancers registered in our county during the same period according to the Swedish Cancer Registry (28). Eighteen of the 23 cancer cases were diagnosed in the group of patients who did not receive any type of follow-up and 5 in the group followed up by physical examination, endoscopy, cytology, and biopsy (Table 23-2).

Gastroscopy was undertaken in patient no. 15, who joined the follow-up scheme on his own initiative, and biopsy revealed carcinoma that proved to be intramucosal in the total gastrectomy specimen. All other cancers were advanced, and metastasis was present in 13 cases. Carcinoma was poorly differentiated in 10 cases and of the signet-ring type in 3. In two cases typing and grading of the carcinoma were not feasible. The stoma was the site of carcinoma either exclusively or together with adjacent parts of the remnant in 12 cases. Almost all the gastric remnant was infiltrated with carcinoma in two cases (Figure 23–4. Compare with Figure 23–5.).

The interval between the date of operation and the diagnosis of carcinoma in the resected stomach ranged from 13 to 49 years, with an average of 25.3 years. However, the mean interval varied according to the age of the patient at the time of operation, being 32, 26, and 20 years for those operated on at 39 years or younger, between 40 and 49 years, and 50 years or older, respectively (Table 23-5). Apart from the three cases discovered at autopsy and the only postoperative mortality, ten inoperable patients died 1 to 17 months after diagnosis of the disease. Two patients are still alive for periods varying from 5 months to 8 years after the operation at the end of the study.

(Text continues on page 300)

Table 23-4. Summary of the Clinical, Histological, and Follow-up Data of 23 Cases of Carcinoma in the Resected Stomach

Patient	Sex	Initial Disease	Operation Year	Operation Type	Age at Operation (years)	Presenting Symptoms	Histology	Site of Ca	Site of Met	Age at Ca Discovery (years)	Outcome
1. K.A.	M	DU	1927	AC, no EA	27	Weight loss, vomiting	Well-diff. adenoCa	Lesser curve, stoma	Pancreas, liver, omentum	76	Died 10 months after diagnosis
2. T.A.	F	GU	1935	AC, no EA	42	Weight loss, dyspepsia, vomiting	AdenoCa	Distal part of stomach remnant with stomal stenosis	Unknown	88	Died 3 months after diagnosis
3. T.L.	F	GU	1938	RC, no EA	39	Anemia, occult bleeding	Well-diff. adenoCa	Greater curve, stoma	Liver, pancreas	80	Died 6 months after diagnosis
4. H.W.	F	DU	1943	AC, no EA	38	Anemia, nausea	Mod. diff. adenoCa	Lesser curve near the stoma	None	75	Alive 26 months after operation
5. B.K.	M	GU	1948	RC, no EA	45	Anemia	Anaplastic Ca	Stoma	None	64	Died 5 months after operation
6. O.A.	M	GU	1951	RC, no EA	51	Anemia, loss of weight	Ca with lymphoid stroma	Lesser curve	None	74	Alive 8 years after operation
7. J.K.	M	GU	1951	RC, no EA	37	Dumping, anemia, epigastric pain, vomiting, hematemesis, melena	Poorly diff. adenoCa	Greater curve, stoma	Infil of mesocolon	59	Died 17 months after diagnosis
8. V.Ö.	F	GU	1952	AC, no EA	48	Anorexia, diffuse abdominal pain, anemia, loss of weight	Poorly diff. adenoCa	Stoma	Infil of abdominal wall	75	Died 3 months after diagnosis
9. A.A.	M	GU	1953	RC, no EA	43	Anemia, melena	Poorly diff. adenoCa	Stoma	Peritoneum	59	Died 5 months after diagnosis

Table 23-4. (continued)

Patient	Sex	Initial Disease	Operation Year	Operation Type	Age at Operation (years)	Presenting Symptoms	Histology	Site of Ca	Site of Met	Age at Ca Discovery (years)	Outcome
10. B.W.	F	DU	1954	AC, no EA	24	Dyspepsia, loss of weight, pain and tenderness in epigastrium, anemia	Ca with lymphoid stroma	Greater curve, posterior wall	None	65	Died 3 months after diagnosis in lung edema
11. A.L.	M	GU	1955	AC + EA	37	Hematemesis, melena	Mod. diff. adenoCa	Greater curve	Unknown	64	Alive 9 months after operation
12. K.-E.P.	M	DU	1955	AC, no EA 1955; EA and vagotomy 1967	56	Anemia	Poorly diff. adenoCa	Around the stoma (lesser curve)	—	79	Died 5 months after operation
13. S.O.	M	GU	1956	AC, no EA	43	Anemia, ascites, palpable swelling in upper abdomen	Signet-ring-type Ca	Fundus 5 cm proximal to stoma; ulcerated tumor 6 cm	Local lymph nodes, lung, liver, omentum, peritoneum	68	Died 2 months after diagnosis
14. J.G.	M	DU	1956	AC, no EA	37	Acute pancreatitis	Poorly diff. adenoCa	Stoma	None	62	Discovered at autopsy
15. G.O.	M	DU	1956	AC, no EA	43	Epigastric pain, weight loss	Superficial Ca	Stoma	None	68	Alive 15 months after operation
16. G.Z.	M	DU	1956	AC, no EA	54	Abdominal pain, rigidity	Signet-ring Ca	Diffuse in the remnant	Pancreas, spleen, mesentery, small and large intestines, peritoneum	77	Diagnosed at autopsy

Table 23-4. (continued)

Patient	Sex	Initial Disease	Operation Year	Type	Age at Operation (years)	Presenting Symptoms	Histology	Site of Ca	Site of Met	Age at Ca Discovery (years)	Outcome
17. B.E.	M	GU + DU	1956	AC, no EA	50	Anemia, hematemesis	Poorly diff. adenoCa	Stoma, proximal jejunal loop	Local lymph nodes	72	Alive 3.5 years after operation
18. S.N.	M	GU	1956	AC, no EA	50	Repeated hematemesis, melena	Poorly diff. adenoCa (10 × 5 × 2 cm)	Stoma	None	71	Discovered at autopsy
19. K.B.	M	DU	1957	AC, no EA	48	Anorexia, anemia, diffuse abdominal pain, weight loss	Poorly diff. adenoCa (5 × 3.5 cm)	Posterior wall	Local lymph nodes	71	Died 1 year after operation with generalized peritoneal metastases
20. E.C.	M	GU	1959	AC, no EA	54	Anemia subjectively normal	Poorly diff. adenoCa	Stoma, lesser curve	Local lymph nodes	74	Postoperative death owing to suture insufficiency
21. L.S.	M	GU + DU	1963	AC, no EA	56	Anemia	Well-diff. partly papillary Ca	Lesser curve	Omentum, small intestine	72	Died 16 months after diagnosis
22. K.S.	M	DU	1964	AC + EA	60	Loss of weight, pain	Ca	Lesser curve	Unknown	73	Died 1 month after diagnosis
23. E.S.	M	GU	1965	AC, no EA	62	Anemia	Signet-ring-type Ca	Almost all gastric remnant	Local lymph nodes	80	Alive 6 months after operation

Abbreviations: AC, antecolic; Ca, carcinoma; DU, duodenal ulcer; EA, enteroanastomosis; GU, gastric ulcer; Infil, infiltration; Met, metastasis; RC, retrocolic.

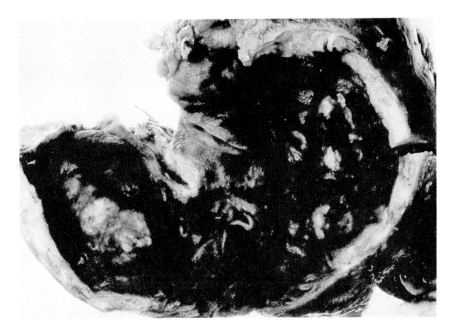

Figure 23-4. The macroscopic appearance of a diffuse carcinoma affecting almost all the gastric remnant in an 80-year-old male 18 years after operation (case no. 23). Note that carcinoma does not extend into the small intestine (*arrows*). This case is to be compared with the case in Figure 23-5.

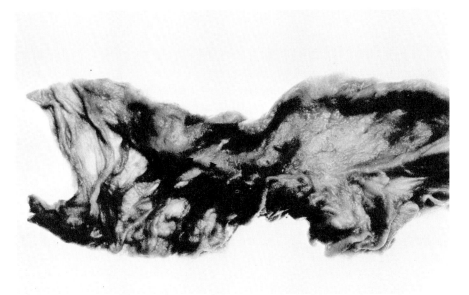

Figure 23-5. The macroscopic appearance of a normal gastric remnant at autopsy of an 89-year-old female 26 years after operation. The arrows point to the gastroenterostomy anastomosis.

Table 23-5. The Interval between Age at Operation and Development of Carcinoma in the Resected Stomach

Age at Operation (years)	No. of Patients	Interval (years)	Average Interval
20–29	2	49, 22	35.5
30–39	5	41, 37, 22, 27, 25	30.4
40–49	7	46, 19, 27, 16, 25, 25, 23	25.6
50–59	7	23, 23, 23, 22, 21, 20, 16	21.1
60–69	2	13, 18	15.5

DISCUSSION

Definition

Carcinoma of the resected stomach (gastric stump or remnant) is a primary disease arising in the gastric remnant at least 5 years after partial gastrectomy, mostly of the Billroth type, for benign disease. This period of time is presumably long enough to rule out the possibility of overlooked or misdiagnosed gastric cancer and the existence of concomitant benign and malignant gastric disease at the time of surgery. A lapse of 10 years has also been recommended (29), but most workers in the field agree to 5 years.

The Value of Review

All original histologic slides of resections performed for benign and malignant disease during the period of study should be reviewed. The value of review is exemplified by the present work in which the original diagnosis was changed in two cases. A very limited number of cases is implicated in such studies, especially when investigating the incidence of carcinoma prospectively, and the addition or exclusion of a few cases may affect the outcome dramatically.

Histopathologic and Diagnostic Considerations

In patients examined by gastroscopy and forceps biopsy, no stomach was completely normal in 63 mostly asymptomatic B-I and B-II gastrectomies (30) and 56 symptomatic B-II patients (31). However, in larger series of patients, normal mucosa was reported in 0.9 (20) to 7.1 (32) percent of patients. In our material the gastric mucosa was normal in 6.2 and 17.1 percent on endoscopic and histologic examinations, respectively. This discrepancy can be due to biopsies not being representative in some cases or to the absence of histological changes in biopsies from mucosa thought to be abnormal on endoscopy. This has been confirmed in a study on erosions to be published elsewhere.

There is general agreement upon the development of mucosal changes in the gastric remnant after gastroenterostomy and partial gastrectomy for benign disease (15, 20, 21, 32–34). The frequent occurence of chronic gastritis with varying degrees of atrophy, intestinal metaplasia, lipid islands, and cystic dilatation of glands has been described 3 to 30 years postoperatively. Peitsch and Becker (25) reported a higher incidence (64 percent) of severe chronic gastritis with or without intestinal metaplasia of gastric remnants after resection for gastric ulcer, the corresponding figure being 32 percent in case of resection for duodenal ulcer. However, Janunger et al. (34) found that partial gastrectomy in duodenal ulcer patients causes a marked increase in inflammatory and other mucosal changes to the same extent as in patients operated on for gastric ulcer. Late postoperatively no correlation could be made between the mucosal changes and factors such as age, sex, type of ulcer, and operative procedure.

Compared with controls, duodenal ulcer patients were found to develop postoperatively significantly more mucosal changes, including epithelial dysplasia around the gastroenterostomy (35). The frequency of dysplasia varied in the literature between 8.5 (18) and 28.6 (31) percent for slight dysplasia, 2.8 (18) and 4.5 (17) percent for moderate dysplasia, and 0.9 (17) and 15.3 (36) percent for severe dysplasia. In our material dysplasia was present in 56 of 227 (24.7 percent) cases—17.6 percent slight, 5.7 percent moderate, and 1.3 percent severe. Follow-up was conducted in 31 cases in which dysplasia regressed in 77.4 percent, was stationary in 12.9 percent, and progressed in 9.7 percent (Table 23-3). Progression was from slight to moderate dysplasia in two cases and to cancer in one. No progression was noted in 3 cases of severe dysplasia among 40 patients followed up for 3 years by Stokkeland et al. (37). Although slight dysplastic changes were quite numerous, moderate and severe dysplasias were present in a few cases but occurred twice as often as in a control group matched for age (33).

It was suggested that patients with enteroanastomosis are less prone to develop dysplasia as they are subjected less to bile reflux than those without enteroanastomosis (33). However, no significant difference in the histological findings was seen in patients with or without visible reflux (15). So far, the cases involved in the study of dysplastic changes are too few and the periods of follow-up too short to justify any objective judgment about the premalignant potential or fate of dysplasia. Such information is of great importance if any decisions are to be made concerning the frequency of follow-up and the management of patients with resected stomachs. For the individual patient, the presence of dysplasia in biopsies constituted a weak predictor for the development of cancer in the only study with the longest available follow-up of 7 years (19).

The mucosal changes including dysplasia and carcinoma are often located in the stoma and usually extend toward the posterior wall near the afferent loop and the cephalic part of the jejunum (25, 38, 39). The anastomosis line to the small intestine seems to act as a barrier against the infiltrating growth of gastric remnant carcinoma (25, 40). It is therefore advisable in prospective follow-up studies of patients with operated stomachs to take most of the biopsy specimens from the stoma and its surroundings. Biopsies from the afferent and efferent loops of the anastomosis had no diagnostic value in our experience.

A large number of biopsies, varying from 6 (34) to 20 (20, 41), has been recommended for the early discovery of premalignant and malignant changes. This has been motivated by the great variation in the extent and distribution of the mucosal lesions and their multifocality (20, 30, 34), but it has to be weighed against the risk of bleeding, which is not negligible in these patients. One of our patients needed blood transfusions because of serious bleeding after forceps biopsy. It has also to be emphasized that taking many biopsies is decisive not only for the sake of increasing the diagnostic accuracy but also for planning the extent of operation and whether the entire gastric remnant should be removed.

Endoscopy alone is not sensitive enough for the discovery of early cancers or premalignant lesions. Our only superficial carcinoma and four of the cases in the series of Huibregtse et al. (36) were not endoscopically suspected, and in none of the cancer cases reported by Schrumpf et al. (20) were the endoscopic appearances of the mucosa interpreted as malignant. The signs and symptoms are not conclusive in this respect, as a great number of patients with resected stomachs are usually symptomatic; but in advanced cases, bleeding, anemia, and weight loss are alarming symptoms.

It has been suggested that brush cytology be routinely used in the study of patients with resected stomachs (41, 42). It is widely accepted that brush cytology in combination with biopsy increases the yield of positive findings when investigating gastric carcinoma. In our experience it is preferable to take cytology before biopsy in case bleeding is caused by the latter if done first. The low diagnostic accuracy of the roentgen examination for the detection of carcinoma of the resected stomach has been commented on by many authors. This is due mainly to the difficulty of the interpretation of X-ray findings caused by the close similarity between benign postoperative changes and cancer. The relevant literature was reviewed by Feldman and Seaman (43), who discussed the difficulties liable to be encountered in the roentgenological diagnosis of various lesions in the resected stomach. However, they concluded that a knowledgeable radiologist, who is familiar with this entity, should be able to make a correct diagnosis in every case.

Etiopathogenetic Considerations

The etiology of carcinoma of the resected stomach, like gastric carcinoma in general, is still obscure. However, some etiopathogenetic factors have been suspected to predispose specific patient groups to cancer. In the following an attempt is made to answer the question of if there are any specific B-II patient groups at risk. The following factors are discussed: age, sex, the initial disease, and the type of gastric operation.

The average age of patients at the time of cancer diagnosis in our series was almost 72 years, which is on the high end of a scale ranging from 42.5 (15) to 73 (44) years, with 66 years as the most frequently cited figure for B-II-operated patients (8, 44–47). This average corresponds to the usual age incidence of gastric cancer irrespective of whether gastroenterostomy, partial gastrectomy, or any other surgical procedure has been carried out. If gastric surgery is to be considered a risk condition, one should expect cancer to develop at an earlier age, as is the case in patients with long-standing ulcerative colitis.

The older the patient at the time of operation, the shorter is the interval between the operation and cancer diagnosis (Table 23-5). The average interval was almost 32, 23.5, and 15.5 years in the age groups of 20 to 39, 40 to 59, and 60 to 69 years, respectively. Similar trends were reported earlier (16, 19, 25, 47). The average interval for all our cancer cases was 25.3 years—somewhat shorter than the longest average of 28.5 years reported by Terjesen and Erichsen (47). In most reports the average interval varied from 20 to 25 years.

There is statistical evidence that males who have undergone resection for benign ulcer disease more than 11 years previously constitute a risk group (16). The predominance of males in any collection of patients with duodenal ulcer makes this evidence difficult to confirm and was not confirmed in other series. Cancer in the above-mentioned study (16) was exclusively in patients operated on for duodenal ulcer. In our series the ratio of cancers arising in males and females was 3.6:1, nearly equal to the ratio of males and females in the whole study.

It has been repeatedly claimed that resection for gastric ulcer implies a greater risk for later development of carcinoma in the gastric remnant than resection for duodenal ulcer (6, 12). This is based on the assumption that the mucosa in which a gastric ulcer develops is also cancer prone. However, many studies do not lend support to this claim (2, 11, 48). The literature pertaining to these questions was reviewed by Janunger et al. (34) who supported the idea that stump cancer is frequently reported with the same frequency independent of operative ulcer disease.

A relevant question to be asked here is: Do results of experimental studies support the idea of a possible risk associated with any of these factors? Langhans et al. (49, 50) critically reviewed recent experimental results of carcinogenesis studies in the operated stomach with and without resection and found their results highly conflicting. Their own experimental assay was designed to elucidate the pathogenetic influence of the surgical trauma as such, the duodenogastric reflux, and carcinogen application. They concluded that carcinomas may arise in the operated stomach with or without the application of chemical carcinogens. The number of carcinomas was found to rise in proportion with the intensity of the duodenogastric reflux resulting from the respective operative procedures, and the superiority of B-II resection with gastroenterostomy following the Roux-en-y method was emphasized. On the other hand, Meister et al. (24) did not find justification to accuse any single factor, such as intestinal reflux, carcinogens, or different surgical techniques, of promoting cancer.

It seems, therefore, that age at operation is the most decisive factor and that carcinoma arising in the resected stomach, like gastric carcinoma in general, is age dependent and occurs after a relatively longer interval in younger than older patients operated on for benign conditions irrespective of sex, the nature of the initial disease and the type of gastric operation.

Epidemiologic Considerations

Carcinoma of the resected stomach has been reported extensively in the European literature, especially from Scandinavia, Germany, and England. Sporadic reports have appeared in the American literature (23, 43, 44, 46, 51), but this entity is seldomly reported from Japan (52) in spite of the high frequency of gastric carcinoma in that country.

If the surgery were an important risk factor for the development of carcinoma in the resected stomach, the incidence ought to be increased in every country.

The Incidence of Carcinoma in the Resected Stomach

There are conflicting reports on the incidence of carcinoma developing in the resected stomach following gastrectomy for benign disease. No cancer was detected in relatively small series of patients (55 to 196) followed up for periods varying from 5 to 30 years (30, 32, 33). No increase in incidence was suggested by some authors (2, 8, 11), whereas others (5, 53) reported that it was lower than the incidence of gastric carcinoma in the general population. Incidences varying from 2 to 13 percent were reported (4, 6, 13–15, 20) from many countries. However, it is difficult to compare these results, as the frequency of gastric carcinoma is subjected to geographical variations. Marked differences are also observed in incidences reported from the same country, as in the cases of England, Holland, Norway, and Sweden (Table 23–6). These differences are possibly due to variations in the number and selection of patients as well as in methods of study and statistical analysis.

The incidence of carcinoma, after the exclusion of cases operated on outside our county, was 0.8 percent (2 of 237 patients) in the material operated on from September 1957 to September 1959, 2.3 percent (5 of 222 patients) in the group of patients followed up by physical examination, endoscopy, cytology, and biopsy, and 7.1 percent (20 of 283 patients) in all patients included in the study. This clearly illustrates how selection can dramatically affect cancer frequency in any material that does not take into account the vast majority, if not all, of the patients operated on. The number of patients lost to follow-up in the prospective studies was often high and amounted to 22.9, 70.8, 57.6, 62.4, 71.9, and 74.3 percent in series published by Domellöf et al. (15), Huibregtse et al. (36), Ewerth et al. (17), Farrands et al. (18), Savage and Jones (30), and Schrumpf et al. (20), respectively.

Two methods of assessing cancer incidence have been adopted. The first relates the number of carcinomas developing in the resected stomach to the overall number of gastrectomies performed for benign disease during the same period retrospectively or prospectively. Retrospective studies are based on autopsy results, clinical outcome, or a combination of both (6, 8, 9, 12, 14). In prospective studies follow-up of patients is conducted either by physical examination and/or interview (54) or by this together with gastroscopy, cytology, and biopsy (15, 17–20, 30). The second method compares the number of partially

Table 23-6. The Frequency of Carcinoma of the Resected Stomach in
Studies from Four Countries

References	Type of Study	No. of Patients (% of Total)	Follow-Up Interval (years)	No. of Cancers (Incidence)
England				
Savage and Jones (30) (Bristol)	Prospective, endoscopy	63 (28%)	15–27	None
Clark et al. (54) (London)	Prospective, annual interview	225 (86.5%)	22–27	1 (0.44%)
Farrands et al. (18) (Nottingham)	Prospective, endoscopy	71 (37.6%)	15–35	2 (2.8%)
Holland				
Huibregtse et al. (36) (Amsterdam)	Prospective, endoscopy	535 (29.2%)	15–46	11 (2.0%)
Welvaart and Warnsinck (53) (Leiden)	Prospective, clinical	257 (97.0%)	Minimum 26	5 (1.9%)
Norway				
Helsingen and Hillestad (6) (Oslo)	Retrospective, mortality	229 (75.6%)	8–28	11 (4.8%)
Schrumpf et al. (20) (Oslo)	Prospective, endoscopy	108 (25.7%)	20–25	4 (3.7%)
Sweden				
Krause (9) (Uppsala)	Retrospective, mortality	361 (94.0%)	23–50	28 (7.8%)
Domellöf et al. (15) (Umeå)	Prospective, endoscopy; retrospective, mortality	354 (77.1%)	17–20	7 (2.0%)
Ewerth et al. (17) (Stockholm)	Prospective, endoscopy; retrospective, mortality	241 (42.4%)	22–26	2 (0.8%)
Eriksson (19) (Lund)	Retrospective, mortality	1,403 (89.1%)	19–49	24 (1.7%)
	Prospective, endoscopy	357 (44.8%)	19–26	22 (6.2%)

gastrectomized patients in collections of persons suffering from gastric cancer with the expected number of gastrectomized patients in a matched control population (2, 11, 13). Incidences calculated according to this method in most of the published series range from 1 to 3 percent (8, 12, 13, 22, 46, 55). The only strictly controlled retrospective study based on autopsy so far was carried out in Norway by Stalsberg and Taksdal (14). They found that the risk of gastric cancer was about five times higher for previous gastrectomies among patients dying with gastric cancer as compared with noncancer matched controls. In Finland Kivilaakso et al. (8) using a similar study design concluded that the risk of cancer in the gastric remnant was not significantly increased as compared with the normal unoperated population. The risk was even found to be lower in resected than in unoperated stomachs in general (24).

The various methods used to calculate the incidence of carcinoma of the resected stomach have been criticized in some recent publications (53, 54, 56). The frequency of such cancers in a group of cases of gastric carcinoma does not represent the real incidence of this condition. On the other hand, comparison of the number of cancers of the resected stomach with the number of resections performed during a certain period of time can be an expression of the variety of patients registered in the files of a clinic or an institution. Other factors contributing to the skepticism are the absence of cancer registries in many countries, the scarcity of properly controlled studies, the limited number of patients involved, and the high percentage of those lost to follow-up, leading to incalculable selection factors. The problem of retrieving the original slides for histopathologic review has been mentioned earlier. Different use of diagnostic criteria may also complicate the comparison, particularly when evaluating dysplastic lesions and mucosal carcinoma.

The ideal control group should include age- and sex-matched patients conservatively treated for gastric or duodenal disease similar to those treated by surgery. This is a prerequisite for the accurate calculation of the true risk, if any, related to gastric resection. An extensive review of the literature (57) revealed that the frequency of cancer after B-II resection for gastric ulcer without enteroanastomosis was not greater than in medically treated gastric ulcers. It is estimated that 10 percent of conservatively treated gastric ulcer patients will subsequently develop gastric cancer.

The Ideal Trial Design

The ideal design for the determination of the true incidence and risk of B-II gastric resection should be a large enough, prospective, randomized, controlled study. Such a trial should take into consideration if screening for carcinoma in B-II-operated patients reduced mortality as compared with a control group of a both nonscreened and non-operated population. However, the results of such a trial would not be available before a very long time, partly because of the relatively very few patients who undergo surgery nowadays and partly because of the long time lapse before the development of carcinoma. An alternative although much inferior method is to analyze the fate of a large number of patients over a long period of time partly retrospectively and partly prospectively using suitable statistical models to estimate eventual gains in terms of survival. One should remember that these patients usually represent an older age group among whom repeated endoscopy can be unpopular and a gastric operation for dysplasia or cancer a great hazard.

Size of the Problem

In a population survey undertaken in the London area in 1951, it was found that 1.1 percent of all people over the age of 45 years had previously undergone surgery for peptic ulcer (12). Hellers et al. (58) estimated the number of risk patients living in Stockholm to be 10,000, constituting 1.6 percent of the total population, which, if reflected on the whole of Sweden, should mean about 130,000 patients. If these patients are to be screened according to the model tried in the northern city Umeå (15, 59), 20,000 endoscopy examinations should be needed annually. This is clearly an impossible aim to fulfill. Similar and even greater problems exist for other countries. The cost will be prohibitive.

All workers in the field agree that the prognosis of carcinoma of the resected stomach is extremely poor once symptoms start to appear. Furthermore, advocates of the screening of gastrectomized patients claim that the prognosis of carcinoma arising in the resected stomach is poorer than gastric cancer in general, and that the only way to improve this is to detect malignancy at a stage when curative resection is still possible. Eriksson (19) found that the 5-year survival rate after surgical treatment for advanced cancer in the operated stomach is similar to that of gastric cancer in the general population. Two questions should be answered before proceeding further: Is discovery of early cancer in the resected stomach possible? Would discovery of precancer or cancer at an early stage in the resected stomach prolong survival?

The detection of early carcinoma in the resected stomach is confirmed by most of the prospective studies, using endoscopy, cytology, and biopsy, which have appeared in the literature since 1976 (15, 20, 39, 55). There is no place for screening only by case history–taking, physical examination, or waiting until symptoms start to appear, as suggested by Clark et al. (54). Case history and physical examination can be valuable supplements to the other investigations. As far as the second question is concerned, the final aim of any screening program for carcinoma in general should be to reduce mortality in the screened as compared with the nonscreened patients. According to the only study that investigated this question (19), mortality from gastric cancer did not differ from the expected during a mean follow-up period of 26 years.

Against the background of the high cost of screening, doubtful information about the increased risk, and the fact that screening does not reduce mortality, screening for carcinoma of the resected stomach on a national basis cannot be justified. However, well-designed studies are encouraged to verify or refute current experiences.

Different models and policies have been proposed for the follow-up of persons with resected stomachs. It was suggested that screening should start from 5 (18, 39) to 10 or 15 years postoperatively and should be repeated after periods as short as 6 months, annually, biennially, or every 3 to 5 years (36, 37, 44). Another alternative is to examine the operated population every 3 years from about the age of 50 years onward (56).

On the basis of our results, particularly those dealing with the length of the interval between surgery and cancer development, an individual-oriented follow-up scheme is preferred. The age at operation governs the lapse of time before the screening of any patient is to be started, and 25, 15, and 10 years are thought suitable for the age groups of 20 to 39, 40 to 59, and 60 years or more, respectively.

The frequency of follow-up is to be planned in light of the result of the first examination. If no dysplastic changes are seen, patients are to be reexamined after 7, 5, and 3 years according to which one of the three age groups they belong to. This period is to be shortened to 1 and 2 years if slight and moderate or severe dysplasia are discovered, respectively. The scheme should be tested and eventually modified in accordance with the growing knowledge about the premalignant nature and fate of dysplasia.

SUMMARY

The resected stomach is the site of a wide spectrum of histopathological changes, including gastritis, intestinal metaplasia, glandular abnormalities, dysplasia, and carcinoma. No correlation could be found between the development of carcinoma and mucosal changes or factors like sex, initial disease, and type of gastric operation. Age at operation is the most decisive factor, as carcinoma arises after a relatively longer interval in younger than older patients, the average age being similar to the usual age incidence of gastric carcinoma in general.

The knowledge gathered about mucosal dysplasia in the resected stomach is too scant to allow judgment about its premalignant potential or fate. No statistically convincing evidence is so far available as to the increased cancer risk in gastrectomized patients. Screening of these patients with gastroscopy and forceps biopsy has not shown favorable effects in terms of the reduction of mortality in gastric carcinoma.

New, well-designed screening trials are needed to settle this important question, but the screening of B-II-gastrectomized patients on a national basis cannot be justified against the background of the current state of knowledge.

ACKNOWLEDGMENT

Endoscopy was carried out by the following colleagues, to whom I am indebted: Dick Aronson, Olle Björklund, Kjell Furugård, Mikulas Hradsky, Ulf Hållmarker, Åke Kjellmert, Göran Perers, Curt Tysk, Jan Ulfberg, and Maria Wikander.

The assistance of the technical and secretarial staff of the Department of Clinical Pathology and Cytology, Falun Hospital, Falun, Sweden, in the preparation of this chapter is greatly appreciated.

REFERENCES

1. Balfour, D. C. Factors influencing the life expectancy of patients operated on for gastric ulcer. *Ann. Surg.* 76 (1922):405–408.
2. DeJode, L. R. Gastric carcinoma following gastroenterostomy and partial gastrectomy. *Br. J. Surg.* 48 (1961):512–514.
3. Denck, H., and Salzer, G. Die frage der Karzinomgefahrdung des ulkuskranken und magenrestzierten. *Gastroenterologia* 88 (1957):94–109.
4. Griesser, G., and Schmidt, H. Statische erhebungher über die häufigkeit des karzinoms nach magenoperation wegen eines geschwürsleidens. *Med. Welt.* 35 (1964):1836–1840.
5. Hakkiluoto, A. Longterm follow-up study of patients operated on for benign peptic ulcer. *Ann. Chir. Gynaecol. Fenn.* 65 (1976):361–368.
6. Helsingen, N., and Hillestad, L. Cancer development in the gastric stump after partial gastrectomy for ulcer. *Ann. Surg.* 143 (1956):173–179.
7. Hilbe, G., Salzer, G. M., Hussl, H., and Kutschera, H. The incidence of cancer in the gastric remnant after subtotal gastric resection. *Arch. Klin. Chir.* 323 (1968):142–153.
8. Kivilaakso, E., Hakkiluoto, A., Kalima, T. V., and Sipponen, P. Relative risk of stump cancer following partial gastrectomy. *Br. J. Surg.* 64 (1977):336–338.
9. Krause, U. Late prognosis after partial gastrectomy for ulcer. *Acta Chir. Scand.* 114 (1958):341–354.
10. Kühlmayer, R., and Rokitansky, O. Das magenstumpfcarzinom als spätproblem der ulcuschirurgie. *Langenbecks Arch. Dtsch. Z. Chir.* 278 (1954):361–364.
11. Liavaag, K. Cancer development in gastric stump after partial gastrectomy for peptic ulcer. *Ann. Surg.* 155 (1962):103–106.
12. Nicholls, J. C. Carcinoma of the stomach following partial gastrectomy for benign gastroduodenal lesions. *Br. J. Surg.* 61 (1974):244–249.
13. Saegesser, F., and Jämes, D. Cancer of the gastric stump after partial gastrectomy (Billroth II principle) for ulcer. *Cancer* 29 (1972):1150–1159.
14. Stalsberg, H., and Taksdal, S. Stomach cancer following gastric surgery for benign conditions. *Lancet* 27 (1971):1175–1177.
15. Domellöf, L., Eriksson, S., and Janunger, K.-G. Carcinoma and possible precancerous changes of the gastric stump after Billroth II resection. *Gastroenterology* 73 (1977):462–468.
16. Domellöf, L., and Janunger, K.-G. The risk for gastric carcinoma after partial gastrectomy. *Am. J. Surg.* 134 (1977):581–584.
17. Ewerth, S., Bergstrand, O., Hellers, G., and Öst, A. The incidence of carcinoma in the gastric remnant after resection for benign ulcer disease. *Acta Chir. Scand. (Suppl.)* 482 (1978):2–5.
18. Farrands, P. A., Blake, J. R. S., Ansell, I. D., Cotton, R. E., and Hardcastle, J. D. Endoscopic review of patients who have had gastric surgery. *Br. Med. J.* 286 (1983):755–758.
19. Eriksson, S. B. S. The operated stomach. M. D. Thesis, Lunds University, 1983.
20. Schrumpf, E., Serck-Hanssen, A., Stadaas, J., Aune, S., Myren, J., and Osnes, M. Mucosal changes in the gastric stump 20–25 years after partial gastrectomy. *Lancet* 2 (1977):467–469.

21. Domellöf, L., Eriksson, S., and Janunger, K.-G. Late precancerous changes and carcinoma of the gastric stump after Billroth I resection. *Am. J. Surg.* 132 (1976):26–31.

22. Gazzola, L. M., and Saegesser, F. Cancer of the gastric stump following operations for benign gastric or duodenal ulcers. *J. Surg. Oncol.* 7 (1975):293–298.

23. Kobayashi, S., Prolla, J. D., and Kirsner, J. B. Late gastric carcinoma developing after surgery for benign conditions. *Dig. Dis.* 15 (1970):905–912.

24. Meister, H., Schlag, P., Weber, E., Bockler, R., and Merkle, P. Frequency of cancerous and precancerous epithelial lesions in the stomach in different models for enterogastric reflux. *Scand. J. Gastroenterol.* 16, Suppl. 67 (1981):165–168.

25. Peitsch, W., and Becker, H. D. Frequency and prognosis of gastric stump cancer. *Front. Gastrointest. Res.* 5 (1979):170 177.

26. Dahlgren, S. The afferent loop syndrome. M. D. Thesis, Uppsala University, 1964.

27. Nagayo, T. Histological diagnosis of biopsied gastric mucosae with special reference to that of borderline lesions. *Gann Monogr. Cancer Res.* 11 (1971): 245–249.

28. National Board of Health. Cancer incidence in Sweden 1969–1979. The Cancer Registry, Stockholm, 1969–79.

29. Pygott, F. Long survival after carcinoma of the stomach. *Gut* 5 (1964):118–125.

30. Savage, A., and Jones, S. Histological appearances of the gastric mucosa 15–27 years after partial gastrectomy. *J. Clin. Pathol.* 32 (1979):179–186.

31. Geboes, K., Rutgeerts, P., Broeckaert, L., Vantrappen, G., and Desmet, V. Histological appearances of endoscopic gastric mucosal biopsies 10–20 years after partial gastrectomy. *Ann. Surg.* 192 (1980):179–182.

32. Graem, N., Fischer, A. B., Hastrup, N., and Poulsen, C. O. Mucosal changes of the Billroth II resected stomach. A follow-up study of patients resected for duodenal ulcer. *Acta. Pathol. Microbiol. Scand.* (A) 89 (1981):227–234.

33. Borchard, F., Mittelstaedt, A., and Kieker, R. Incidence of epithelial dysplasia after partial gastric resection. *Pathol. Res. Pract.* 164 (1979):282–293.

34. Janunger, K.-G., Domellöf, L., and Eriksson, S. The development of mucosal changes after gastric surgery for ulcer disease. *Scand. J. Gastroenterol.* 13 (1978):217–223.

35. Saukkonen, M., Sipponen, P., and Kekki, M. The morphology and dynamics of the gastric mucosa after partial gastrectomy. *Ann. Clin. Res.* 13 (1981):156–158.

36. Huibregtse, K., Offerhaus, J., Verhoeven, T., de Boer, J., v d Stadt, J., and Tytgat, G. N. Endoscopic screening for malignancy in the gastric remnant. *Acta Endosc.* 11 (1981):171–173.

37. Stokkeland, M., Schrumpf, E., Serck-Hanssen, A., Myren, J., Osnes, M., and Stadaas, J. Incidence of malignancies of the Billroth II operated stomach. A prospective follow-up. *Scand. J. Gastroenterol.* 16, Suppl. 67 (1981):169–171.

38. Hammar, E. The localisation of precancerous changes and carcinoma after previous gastric operation for benign condition. *Acta Pathol. Microbiol. Scand.* 84 (1976):495–507.

39. Langer, S., and Peters, H. The superficial carcinoma in the resected stomach. *Act. Chir.* 12 (1977):377–382.

40. Schlag, P., Merkle, P., and Meister, H. The local tumor distribution of carcinoma and carcinoma recurrence in the operated stomach. *Med. Welt.* 28 (1977):810–812.

41. Osnes, M., Løtveit, T., Myren, J., and Serck-Hanssen, A. Early gastric carcinoma in patients with a Billroth II partial gastrectomy. *Endoscopy* 9 (1977):45–49.

42. Lobello, R., and D'Armiento, M. Cancer of the gastric stump. *Minerva Chir.* 33 (1978):1163–1170.

43. Feldman, F., and Seaman, W. B. Primary gastric stump cancer. *Am. J. Roentgenol.* 115 (1972):257–267.

44. Klarfeld, J., and Resnick, G. Gastric remnant carcinoma. *Cancer* 44 (1979):1129–1133.

45. Dahm, K., Eichfuss, H. P., and Koch, W. Cancer of the gastric stump after Billroth II resection. The influence of gastroenteric anastomosis. *Front. Gastrointest. Res.* 5 (1979):164–169.

46. Dougherty, S. H., Foster, C. A., and Eisenberg, M. M. Stomach cancer following gastric surgery for benign disease. *Arch. Surg.* 117 (1982):294–297.

47. Terjesen, T., and Erichsen, H. G. Carcinoma of the gastric stump after operation for benign gastroduodenal ulcer. *Acta Chir. Scand.* 142 (1976):256–260.

48. Pack, G. T., and Banner, R. L. The late development of gastric carcinoma after gastroenterostomy and gastrectomy for peptic ulcer and benign pyloric stenosis. *Surgery* 44 (1958):1024–1033.

49. Langhans, P., Heger, R. A., Hohenstein, J., Schlake, W., and Bünte, H. Operation sequel carcinoma of the stomach. Experimental studies of surgical techniques with or without resection. *World J. Surg.* 5 (1981):595–605.

50. Langhans, P., Heger, R. A., Hohenstein, J., and Bünte, H. Gastric stump carcinoma. New aspects deduced from experimental results. *Scand. J. Gastroenterol.* 16, Suppl. 67 (1981):161–164.

51. Morgenstern, L., Yamakawa, T., and Seltzer, D. Carcinoma of the gastric stump. *Am. J. Surg.* 125 (1973):29–38.

52. Tsukushi, S., Kato, A., Nakajima, M., Yoshida, R., Fukuchi, S., and Ikenaga, T. Carcinoma development in the gastric remnant after surgery for benign lesions. *Jpn. J. Gastroenterol.* 64 (1967):1033–1034.

53. Welvaart, K., and Warnsinck, H. M. The incidence of carcinoma of the gastric remnant. *J. Surg. Oncol.* 21 (1982):104–106.

54. Clark, C. G., Ward, M. W. N., McDonald, A. M., and Tovey, F. I. The incidence of gastric stump cancer. *World J. Surg.* 7 (1983):236–240.

55. Eberlein, T. J., Lorenzo, F. V., and Webster, M. W. Gastric carcinoma following operation for peptic ulcer disease. *Ann. Surg.* 187 (1978):251–256.

56. Hermanek, P., and Riemann, J. F. The operated stomach—still a precancerous condition? *Endoscopy* 14 (1982):113–114.

57. Peitsch, W., and Becker, H. D. What is certain about the pathogenesis and frequency of primary carcinoma of gastric stump? *Chirurg.* 50 (1979):33–38.

58. Hellers, G., Ewerth, S., and Öst, O. Cancer i ventrikelstumpen efter tidigare resektion för benignt ulcus. *Läkartidningen* 78 (1981):3392–3394.

59. Domellöf, L. Cancer efter ulcuskirurgi-realistisk uppföljning behövs. *Läkartidningen* 80 (1983):28–29.

VIII CONCLUSION

24 PRECURSORS OF GASTRIC CANCER: CURRENT ASSESSMENT

S.-C. Ming

Precursors of gastric cancer can be separated into two categories: precancerous conditions and precancerous lesions (1) or changes (2). Precancerous conditions are disease entities that have an increased risk for gastric cancer. Precancerous lesions or changes are pathological tissue changes from which cancer may develop. Most kinds of precancerous conditions have been known for many years, but the understanding of precancerous lesions is relatively recent. As better investigative methods have been developed and as more data have accumulated, new concepts have emerged. The information presented in this book focuses on the current views on many aspects of these problems. These views are summarized as follows.

EPITHELIAL DYSPLASIA

Dysplasia of the gastric epithelium is a precancerous lesion. It has been variously classified according to the grades of cellular and architectural abnormalities of the epithelium. The precancerous significance of dysplasia has usually been judged according to its association with cancer. Recently, advances in endoscopic biopsy have made it possible to follow the lesion and observe its evolution. Based on a few studies of this nature, it was recommended by the Pathology Panel of the International Study Group on Gastric Cancer to limit the usage of the term "dysplasia" to moderate to severe degrees of abnormality and to place the mild lesions, which are not considered to have precancerous significance, in the category of severe or atypical hyperplasia (Chapter 2). Examples of tissue changes in these lesions are given in Chapters 2 to 5.

Data from follow-up studies are presented in Chapters 4 to 7. These studies document the progression of severely dysplastic epithelium to cancer. However, follow-up studies have been initiated only recently. The discovery of cancer within months or even 3 years of initially benign biopsy may still mean a phenomenon of association rather than causation. Then there is the question of the reversibility of dysplastic epithelium to normal or merely hyperplastic. Further studies along these lines are clearly essential. Guidelines for such studies are proposed by several authors (Chapters 5 to 8).

CHRONIC GASTRITIS

That chronic gastritis is a precancerous condition has been reaffirmed. In terms of premalignant potential, it should be classified according to the etiological and topographical patterns of the disease (Chapter 9), the degree of epithelial atrophy (Chapter 10), and the presence or absence of metaplastic changes (Chapter 11). Distribution of the lesion at the lesser curvature and transitional zone of the stomach, severe atrophy, and metaplasia favor cancer development. Thus, these factors must be documented and taken into account, particularly in prospective studies.

INTESTINAL METAPLASIA

Extensive metaplasia is common in chronic atrophic gastritis. Therefore, these two conditions are often simultaneously considered in terms of their precancerous nature. However, focal metaplasia may be seen without significant atrophy, and the atrophic mucosa is not always metaplastic. Furthermore, metaplasia also occurs in conditions other than atrophic gastritis. The role of metaplasia in carcinogenesis, therefore, deserves consideration according to its own merits.

In recent years, there has been renewed interest in intestinal metaplasia because of the realization of its heterogeneous nature and the possible variance in the carcinogenic role played by its different forms. The complexity of the metaplastic epithelium is discussed in Chapters 12 and 13. Two specific features appear to be more closely related to gastric carcinogenesis than the others: the incomplete form of metaplasia and sulfomucin secretion by the metaplastic mucous cells (Chapters 14 and 15). On the other hand, the importance of metaplasia as a precancerous lesion has been questioned (Chapters 8, 12, and 16), although gastric cancers are frequently composed of intestinal-type cells. It is apparent that both carcinogenic and benign injuries can initiate the metaplastic processes. Animal experiments have shown that carcinogens can cause both cancer and metaplasia as coincidental but independent lesions, and that metaplasia is not a prerequisite for cancer development. Application of these views to the human is supported by the fact that human gastric cancers with prominent metaplasia in the background mucosa are composed predominantly of intestinal-type cells, but the reverse relationship is not as evident. Because of this association intestinal metaplasia may be viewed as a marker of intestinal-type cancer, particularly if the metaplasia is incomplete and sulfomucin is present. The presence of fetal antigen appears to have a similar significance (Chapter 17).

That cancer can develop in the metaplastic epithelium is unquestioned. It is not clear, however, if cancer develops preferentially in the metaplastic epithelium, and, if so, what type of cancer. Prospective studies by endoscopic biopsy would be useful in solving this problem.

POLYPS

The subtypes of gastric polyps and their relationship to cancer are discussed in Chapter 18. Although there is a general agreement on the nature of polyps, some disagreements remain. For instance, questions have been raised as to whether the flat adenomas are true neoplasms or only protruded dysplastic lesions (Chapters 19 and 20). Flat adenoma has been called simply a borderline lesion by some investigators because it may become malignant (Chapters 3 and 8), whereas most pathologists would apply this term to a lesion whose cellular features lie between benignity and malignancy and whose true identity is uncertain. In any case, there is no question about the dysplastic nature and the malignant potential of these lesions.

The hyperplastic polyp of the stomach has been considered to be nonneoplastic and not to have premalignant potential. Recently, however, malignant change in the hyperplastic polyp has been documented. Malignancy occurs through the stage of either dysplastic or adenomatous change. Although such cases are few, their existence can no longer be denied.

CHRONIC GASTRIC ULCER

The importance of chronic gastric ulcer as a precancerous condition has been downgraded. This change of view is particularly evident in Japan, where the incidence of the deeply ulcerated type of early gastric cancer has been drastically reduced. Gastroscopic biopsies have revealed a high rate of missed diagnoses for cancer, on one hand, and the ability of the malignant ulcer to heal, on the other. Both of these findings focus on the importance of accurate diagnosis at the initial examination. These aspects are discussed in Chapters 21 and 22. A further decrease in the incidence of ulcer-promoted cancer may be anticipated as the medical management of ulcer and the diagnostic accuracy of carcinoma improve.

POSTRESECTION GASTRIC STUMP

The development of carcinoma in the gastric stump many years after resection has been repeatedly documented. This phenomenon is critically examined in Chapter 23. It is noted that stump carcinomas develop at the usual age for gastric cancer in general, raising the question of if the postresection state is really precancerous. Further studies are needed to clarify this question. A schedule for follow-up study is suggested.

CONCLUSION

In summary, a careful examination of the role of various conditions in gastric carcinogenesis has raised many questions as to their true precancerous nature. These questions are important: On the one hand, they dissipate the premalignant importance for some of these conditions that has been taken for granted but that was founded on uncritical data bases; on the other, they emphasize the areas of investigation that are important not only for data analysis but also for the management of individual patients. Many practical considerations are offered for clinical follow-up and evaluation studies.

Epithelial dysplasia emerges as the undisputed yardstick or warning signal for anticipated malignant change. Dysplasia can be evaluated only by pathological examination, which can now be used as a monitoring device by repeated gastroscopic biopsies. The proposed criteria (Chapter 2) for the diagnosis of dysplasia as a precancerous lesion should diminish unnecessary concern when the abnormalities are insignificant as well as enhance the necessary care when the abnormalities are severe.

Chronic gastritis and intestinal metaplasia are related mainly to the intestinal type of gastric cancer, since they are common features in the background mucosa for this type of cancer. Dysplasia is also likely to be present in this situation. On the other hand, these changes are not prominently associated with the diffusely infiltrative carcinoma, the prototype of which is the signet-ring cell type. In fact, both the cell origin and the histogenetic processes of this type of cancer remain uncertain. There are indications that it arises from the neck mucous cells (3,4). A similar observation was made experimentally (5).

There are at least three modes of histological presentation by the residual glands in the mucosa infiltrated by a diffuse carcinoma: The glands are relatively normal; they are infiltrated by the cancer cells (Figure 24-1); or they are dysplastic (Figure 24-2). Metaplasia and dys-

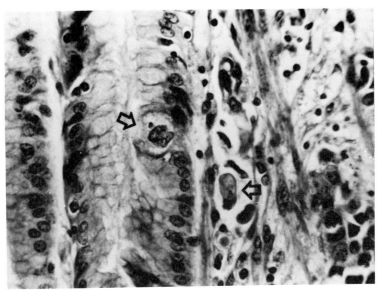

Figure 24-1.   Individual cancer cells (*arrows*) are present in the stroma and an essentially normal gland in a case of diffuse carcinoma. H&E stain. ×600.

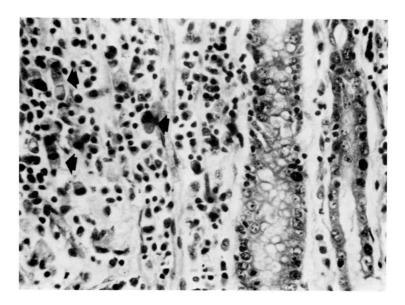

Figure 24-2.   Several cancer cells (*arrows*) are present in the lamina propria on the left. The glands on the right are dysplastic. H&E stain. × 375.

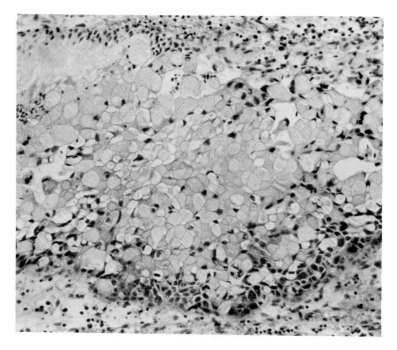

Figure 24-3.   Globoid cells in a dilated foveola. Normal cells are shown at the upper left corner. The outline of the upper right border of the gland is disrupted. There are no infiltrating cancer cells in the stroma. H&E stain. × 160.

plasia are seen in only a minority of cases. The presence of cancer cells in an otherwise normal gland would indicate only tumor invasion.

Recently, another type of abnormality, so-called globoid dysplasia, or metaplasia, has been considered to be a possible precursor of signet-ring cell carcinoma (6). In this situation the foveolar mucous cells become globoid with eccentric nuclei and cytoplasm filled with mucin (Figure 24-3). These cells may occupy only one portion of the foveola. The abnormal cells appear to be ballooned-up mucous cells containing mainly sialomucin. Thus, the phenomenon is akin to incomplete intestinal metaplasia. These cells resemble signet-ring cells, and it is conceivable that they are related to diffuse carcinoma or even other types of gastric cancer as well (see Chapter 6). However, they have been seen in the dilated foveolae of hyperplastic polyps where there is no invasive carcinoma nearby. Furthermore, they are rare even in cases of signet-ring cell carcinoma. Further studies are needed to clarify the importance of globoid cells as precancerous.

REFERENCES

1. Morson, B. C., Sobin, L. H., Grundmann, E., Johansen, A., Nagayo, T., and Serck-Hanssen, A. Precancerous conditions and epithelial dysplasia in the stomach. *J. Clin. Pathol.* 33 (1980):711–721.
2. Nagayo, T. Precursors of human gastric cancer: Their frequencies and histological characteristics. In *Pathophysiology of Carcinogenesis in Digestive Organs*, edited by Farber, E., Kawachi, T., Nagayo, T., Sugano, H., Sugimura, T., and Weisburger, J. H. pp. 151–161. Tokyo: University of Tokyo Press, 1977.
3. Yamashiro, K., Suzuki, H., and Nagayo, T. Electron microscopic study of signet-ring cells in diffuse carcinoma of the human stomach. *Virchows Arch. (Pathol. Anat.)* 374 (1977):275–284.
4. Grundmann, E. Histologic types and possible initial stages in early gastric carcinoma. *Beitr. Pathol.* 154 (1975):256–280.
5. Watanabe, H., Hirose, F., Takizawa, S., Terada, Y., Fugii, I., and Ohkita, T. A mode of incipient growth in chemically induced signet ring cell carcinoma of the canine stomach. *Pathol. Res. Pract.* 164 (1979):216–223.
6. Bordi, C. Gastric carcinoma precursors. *Istocitopatologia* 4 (1982):57.

INDEX

Note: (t) = Table.

F
A